THE SCIENCE OF SPORT
Sprinting

Dr Geoffrey K Platt

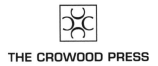

THE CROWOOD PRESS

First published in 2015 by
The Crowood Press Ltd
Ramsbury, Marlborough
Wiltshire SN8 2HR

www.crowood.com

British Library Cataloguing-in-Publication Data
A catalogue record for this book is available from the British Library.

ISBN 978 1 84797 941 4

Typeset by Servis Filmsetting Ltd, Stockport, Cheshire

Printed and bound in India by Replika Press Pvt Ltd

CONTENTS

AUTHORS AND CONTRIBUTORS

Dr Geoffrey K. Platt is an international coach, lecturer and author. He is retained by the International Olympic Committee (IOC), the World Anti-Doping Agency (WADA), the International Weightlifting Federation (IWF) and the International Powerlifting Federation (IPF) to lecture on a wide range of subjects relating to high performance sport. He is a former principal lecturer in Sports Coaching Science.

Professor Morteza Shahbazi Moghaddam is an emeritus professor from Tehran University. He received his PhD from Paris University in Electronics in 1974, but since 1986 he has been involved with biomechanics, and following a sabbatical at the Centre for Aquatic Research at Edinburgh University in 2001, has continued there as a visiting professor, undertaking research and publishing forty-five papers in this domain.

Dr Mohsen Shafizadeh is a senior lecturer in Skill Acquisition and Performance Analysis at Sheffield Hallam University. He is a qualified athletics coach and technical official in Iran; also a BASES-accredited sports scientist and ISPAS-accredited performance analyst.

Dr Gino di Matteo qualified as a physiotherapist in 1985 before completing a Masters in 1994 and a doctorate in 1999. He is currently the Director of Clinical Services for TW1 Physiotherapy Ltd, and lectures to physicians, surgeons and other healthcare professionals. He has been involved with the assessment and management of injured athletes of all levels, including premiership football and rugby, and lectured to medics preparing for the 2012 Olympics, specializing in the biomechanical assessment of musculoskeletal injuries.

Dr Justin Roberts (Senior Lecturer/Researcher specializing in Performance Nutrition and Physiology at Anglia Ruskin University, Cambridge. He is an Accredited Sport and Exercise Physiologist and Chartered Scientist with the British Association of Sport and Exercise Sciences (BASES). Dr Roberts is also an applied nutritionist registered with the British Association of Applied Nutrition and Nutritional Therapy (BANT), the Nutrition Therapy Council (NTC) and the Complementary and Natural Healthcare Council (CNHC).

Professor Dave Collins is the chair and director of the Institute of Coaching and Performance (IcaP). As an applied performance psychologist, Dave has worked with over sixty world and Olympic medallists, plus a number of professional and international athletes in various team sports. In previous careers he served as Performance Director of UK Athletics, as a teacher and teacher educator, and as a director of coaching for various sports and academies.

Dr Andrew Cruickshank is an ex-professional footballer and current chartered sport psychologist who has worked in elite athletics, motor sport, judo, golf, football, rugby, mountain biking and netball. As an academic, Andrew has a PhD in applied sport psychology, has published work in various journals, and contributed to book chapters on high performance sport.

Susan Giblin is a performance scientist, and a researcher at the Institute of Coaching and Performance (ICaP) at UCLan, specializing in psychomotor skill development. She is a certified strength and conditioning specialist (NSCA) with applied coaching experience to Olympic level. She is currently still in training as a sprints athlete.

Tom McNab is a former Principal National Coach for Athletics. As well as coaching British athletics teams, he also worked with the British Olympic bobsleigh team and the England rugby squad at the 1992 World Cup. In that same year Tom was voted British Coach of the Year. Tom now has a successful career as a novelist and motivational public speaker.

Wilf Paish was one of Britain's most successful athletics coaches in a career spanning five decades. As well as being Principal National Coach for Athletics, he also coached many top class athletes, most notably Tessa Sanderson, who won javelin gold at the 1984 Los Angeles Olympics. Wilf died in 2010.

CHAPTER I

AN INTRODUCTION TO THE SCIENCE OF SPRINTING

by Dr Geoffrey K. Platt

This book is about running as fast as is humanly possible. Some of the best sprinters in the world have combined with some of the best coaches and some of the best injury specialists and some of the best sports scientists to review recent work in the area, and to give their best advice on the direction in which sprinting should develop over the next twenty years.

Since the 1880s, sport has become organized, structured and very competitive. Athletes are no longer the only participants in sport who want to be the best in their field: now coaches, administrators, technical officials, even sports doctors devote their lives, night and day, to being as good as they can be.

THE BACKGROUND TO SPORTS SCIENCE

The end of World War II in 1945 saw the formation of the German Democratic Republic (GDR) – East Germany. Sitting in the shadow of the much larger Federal German Republic (FDR) – West Germany – the East Germans were keen to show what they could do, and

that they could compete against their much larger neighbours. They established the best sports-science set-up that the world has ever seen.

In 1981, Australia formed the Australian Institute of Sport (AIS), which has been 'the cradle of Australia's national sports system – one that is recognized the world over for its ability to identify, develop and produce world, Olympic and Paralympic champions'. The Australians showed that sports science research was not limited to Eastern Europe, and also demonstrated what could be achieved in sports performance with strong investment.

In 2002, England started the English Institute of Sport, with similar organizations in each of the other Home Countries, and 'Olympic sports have leapt ahead and are leading the way in the appliance of expertise, and this is down to the breadth of experts they employ, many of whom have been young graduates employed in specific roles.'

In the words of Sir Dave Brailsford, Performance Director of British Cycling, 'Sport science and medicine are inextricably linked to performance and are areas that British Cycling has continued to embrace.'

In this book, leading athletes, coaches, injury specialists and sports scientists will explain the science and medicine that will move sprinting forwards over the next twenty years.

Definition of Terms

No introduction would be complete unless it defines the terms on which it relies:

Science is defined as 'A systematic study using observation, experiment and measurement, of physical and social phenomena, or any specific area involving such a study.'

Sprinting is defined as 'A run of short distance which can be covered at top speed in one continuous effort.'

'Study the past if you would define the future.' – Confucius (551bc–479bc).

Men

100 Metres

The International Olympic Committee (IOC) and the International Association of Athletics Federation (IAAF) recognize three sprinting events for both men and women for outdoor competition: 100 metres, 200 metres and 400 metres.

ATHLETICS – WORLD RECORDS

World records for athletics were first officially recognized by the IAAF in 1913. Initially, records were accepted for ninety-six men's events; this list has been reduced at various times, including the elimination of imperial distances (except the 1 mile), in 1977. From 1977, all records at sprint distances up to 400 metres have only been accepted if timed fully automatically. Prior to that date the best hand-timed results have been listed.

Record	Name	Nationality	Venue	Date
10.6	Donald Lippincott	USA	Stockholm	6 Jul 1912
10.6	Jackson Scholz	USA	Stockholm	16 Sep 1920
10.4	Charles Paddock	USA	Redlands	23 Apr 1921
10.4	Eddie Tolan	USA	Stockholm	8 Aug 1929
10.4	Eddie Tolan	USA	København	25 Aug 1929
10.3	Percy Williams	CAN	Toronto	9 Aug 1930
10.3	Eddie Tolan	USA	Los Angeles	1 Aug 1932
10.3	Ralph Metcalfe	USA	Budapest	12 Aug 1933
10.3	Eulace Peacock	USA	Oslo	6 Aug 1934
10.3	Christiaan Berger	NED	Amsterdam	26 Aug 1934
10.3	Ralph Metcalfe	USA	Osaka	15 Sep 1934
10.3	Ralph Metcalfe	USA	Dairen	23 Sep 1934
10.3	Takayoshi Yoshioka	JPN	Tokyo	15 Jun 1935
10.2	Jesse Owens	USA	Chicago	20 Jun 1936
10.2	Harold Davis	USA	Compton	6 Jun 1941

100 Metres

Record	Name	Nationality	Venue	Date
10.2	Lloyd LaBeach	PAN	Fresno	15 May 1948
10.2	'Barney' Ewell	USA	Evanston	9 Jul 1948
10.2	McDonald Bailey	GBR	Beograd	25 Aug 1951
10.2	Heinz Fütterer	FRG	Yokohama	31 Oct 1954
10.2	Bobby Morrow	USA	Houston	19 May 1956
10.2	Ira Murchison	USA	Compton	1 Jun 1956
10.2	Bobby Morrow	USA	Bakersfield	22 Jun 1956
10.2	Ira Murchison	USA	Los Angeles	29 Jun 1956
10.2	Bobby Morrow	USA	Los Angeles	29 Jun 1956
10.1	Willie Williams	USA	Berlin	3 Aug 1956
10.1	Ira Murchison	USA	Berlin	4 Aug 1956
10.1	Leamon King	USA	Ontario, CA	20 Oct 1956
10.1	Leamon King	USA	Santa Ana	27 Oct 1956
10.1	Ray Norton	USA	San Jose	18 Apr 1959
10.0	Armin Hary	FRG	Zürich	21 Jun 1960
10.0	Harry Jerome	CAN	Saskatoon	15 Jul 1960
10.0	Horacio Esteves	VEN	Caracas	15 Aug 1964
10.0	Bob Hayes	USA	Tokyo	15 Oct 1964
10.0	Jim Hines	USA	Modesto	27 May 1967
10.0	Enrique Figuerola	CUB	Budapest	17 Jun 1967
10.0	Paul Nash	RSA	Krugersdorp	2 Apr 1968
10.0	Oliver Ford	USA	Albuquerque	31 May 1968
10.0	Charlie Greene	USA	Sacramento	20 Jun 1968
10.0	Roger Bambuck	FRA	Sacramento	20 Jun 1968
9.9	Jim Hines	USA	Sacramento	20 Jun 1968
9.9	Ronnie Ray Smith	USA	Sacramento	20 Jun 1968
9.9	Charlie Greene	USA	Sacramento	20 Jun 1968
9.9	Jim Hines	USA	Ciudad de México	14 Oct 1968
9.9	Eddie Hart	USA	Eugene	1 Jul 1972
9.9	Rey Robinson	USA	Eugene	1 Jul 1972
9.9	Steve Williams	USA	Los Angeles	21 Jun 1974
9.9	Silvio Leonard	CUB	Ostrava	5 Jun 1975
9.9	Steve Williams	USA	Siena	16 Jul 1975
9.9	Steve Williams	USA	Berlin	22 Aug 1975
9.9	Steve Williams	USA	Gainesville	27 Mar 1976
9.9	Harvey Glance	USA	Columbia	3 Apr 1976
9.9	Harvey Glance	USA	Baton Rouge	1 May 1976
9.9	Don Quarrie	JAM	Modesto	22 May 1976

100 Metres

Record	Name	Nationality	Venue	Date
Automatic timing:				
9.95	Jim Hines	USA	Ciudad de México	14 Oct 1968
9.93	Calvin Smith	USA	USAF Academy	3 Jul 1983
9.92	Carl Lewis	USA	Seoul	24 Sep 1988
9.90	Leroy Burrell	USA	New York	14 Jun 1991
9.86	Carl Lewis	USA	Tokyo	25 Aug 1991
9.85	Leroy Burrell	USA	Lausanne	6 Jul 1994
9.84	Donovan Bailey	CAN	Atlanta	27 Jul 1996
9.79	Maurice Greene	USA	Athína	16 Jun 1999
9.77	Asafa Powell	JAM	Athína	14 Jun 2005
9.77	Asafa Powell	JAM	Gateshead	11 Jun 2006
9.77	Asafa Powell	JAM	Zürich	18 Aug 2006
9.74	Asafa Powell	JAM	Rieti	9 Sep 2007
9.72	Usain Bolt	JAM	New York	31 May 2008
9.69	Usain Bolt	JAM	Beijing	16 Aug 2008
9.58	Usain Bolt	JAM	Berlin	16 Aug 2009
Annulled by IAAF:				
9.83	Ben Johnson	CAN	Roma	30 Aug 1987

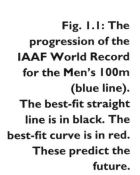

Fig. 1.1: The progression of the IAAF World Record for the Men's 100m (blue line). The best-fit straight line is in black. The best-fit curve is in red. These predict the future.

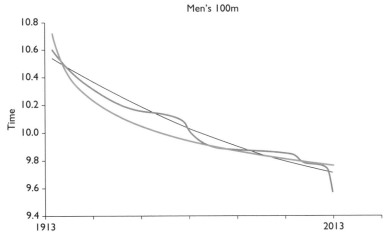

9

200 Metres

y denotes 220 yards time equal to, or better than, the existing metric record

Record	Name	Nationality	Venue	Date
21.2y	William Applegarth	GBR	London	14 Jul 1914
20.6y	Andy Stanfield	USA	Philadelphia	26 May 1951
20.6	Andy Stanfield	USA	Los Angeles	28 Jun 1952
20.6	Thane Baker	USA	Bakersfield	23 Jun 1956
20.6	Bobby Morrow	USA	Melbourne	27 Nov 1956
20.6	Manfred Germar	FRG	Wuppertal	1 Oct 1958
20.6y	Ray Norton	USA	Berkeley	19 Mar 1960
20.6	Ray Norton	USA	Philadelphia	30 Apr 1960
20.5y	Peter Radford	GBR	Wolverhampton	28 May 1960
20.5	Stone Johnson	USA	Palo Alto	2 Jul 1960
20.5	Ray Norton	USA	Palo Alto	2 Jul 1960
20.5	Livio Berruti	ITA	Roma	3 Sep 1960
20.5	Livio Berruti	ITA	Roma	3 Sep 1960
20.5y	Paul Drayton	USA	Walnut	23 Jun 1962
20.3y	Henry Carr	USA	Tempe	23 Mar 1963
20.2y	Henry Carr	USA	Tempe	4 Apr 1964
20.0y	Tommie Smith	USA	Sacramento	11 Jun 1966
19.8	Tommie Smith	USA	Ciudad de México	16 Oct 1968
19.8	Don Quarrie	JAM	Calí	3 Aug 1971
19.8	Don Quarrie	JAM	Eugene	7 Jun 1975
Automatic timing:				
19.83	Tommie Smith	USA	Ciudad de México	16 Oct 1968
19.72	Pietro Mennea	ITA	Ciudad de México	12 Sep 1979
19.66	Michael Johnson	USA	Atlanta	23 Jun 1996
19.32	Michael Johnson	USA	Atlanta	1 Aug 1996
19.30	Usain Bolt	JAM	Beijing	20 Aug 2008
19.19	Usain Bolt	JAM	Berlin	20 Aug 2009

Note that it was not until 1951 that the IAAF first distinguished between records made on a full turn and those marks made on a straight track, which would be c.0.3–0.4 faster. Records were accepted by the IAAF for 200m and 220y on straight tracks until 1975 – the final record (at 220 yards) was 19.5 by Tommie Smith at San Jose on 7 May 1966.

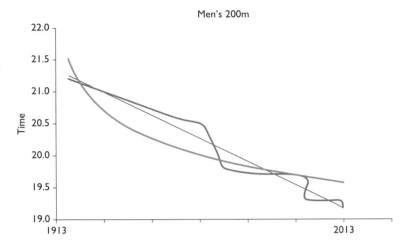

Men's 200m

Fig. 1.2: The progression of the IAAF World Record for the Men's 200m (blue line). The best-fit straight line is in black. The best-fit curve is in red. These predict the future.

400 Metres

y denotes 440 yards time equal to, or better than, the existing metric record

Record	Name	Nationality	Venue	Date
47.8y	Maxie Long	USA	New York (Travers Island)	29 Sep 1910
47.4y	Ted Meredith	USA	Cambridge, MA	27 May 1916
47.0	Bud Spencer	USA	Stanford	12 May 1928
46.4y	Ben Eastman	USA	Stanford	26 Mar 1932
46.2	Bill Carr	USA	Los Angeles	5 Aug 1932
46.1	Archie Williams	USA	Chicago	19 Jun 1936
46.0	Rudolf Harbig	GER	Frankfurt-am-Main	12 Aug 1939
46.0	Grover Klemmer	USA	Philadelphia	29 Jun 1941
46.0y	Herb McKenley	JAM	Berkeley	5 Jun 1948
45.9	Herb McKenley	JAM	Milwaukee	2 Jul 1948
45.8	George Rhoden	JAM	Eskilstuna	22 Aug 1950
45.4	Lou Jones	USA	Ciudad de México	18 Mar 1955
45.2	Lou Jones	USA	Los Angeles	30 Jun 1956
44.9	Otis Davis	USA	Roma	6 Sep 1960
44.9	Carl Kaufmann	FRG	Roma	6 Sep 1960
44.9y	Adolph Plummer	USA	Tempe	25 May 1963
44.9	Mike Larrabee	USA	Los Angeles	12 Sep 1964
44.5	Tommie Smith	USA	San Jose	20 May 1967
44.1	Larry James	USA	Echo Summit	14 Sep 1968
Automatic timing:				
43.86	Lee Evans	USA	Ciudad de México	18 Oct 1968
43.29	Butch Reynolds	USA	Zürich	17 Aug 1988
43.18	Michael Johnson	USA	Sevilla	26 Aug 1999

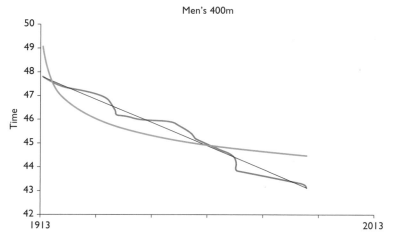

Men's 400m

Fig. 1.3: The progression of the IAAF World Record for the Men's 400m (blue line). The best-fit straight line is in black. The best-fit curve is in red. These predict the future.

Women

Women's records were accepted by the Fédération Sportive Féminine Internationale (FSFI) from its formation in 1921. The FSFI merged with the IAAF in 1936.

100 Metres

Record	Name	Nationality	Venue	Date
13.6	Marie Mejzlíková	TCH	Praha	5 Aug 1922
12.8	Mary Lines	GBR	Paris	20 Aug 1922
12.4	Gundel Wittmann	GER	Braunschweig	22 Aug 1926
12.2	Kinue Hitomi	JPN	Osaka	20 May 1928
12.0	Myrtle Cook	CAN	Halifax	2 Jul 1928
12.2	Betty Robinson	USA	Amsterdam	1 Aug 1928
12.0	Tollien Schuurman	NED	Amsterdam	31 Aug 1930
11.9	Tollien Schuurman	NED	Haarlem	5 Jun 1932
11.9	Stanislawa Walasiewicz	POL	Los Angeles	1 Aug 1932
11.8	Stanislawa Walasiewicz	POL	Poznan	17 Sep 1933
11.7	Stanislawa Walasiewicz	POL	Warszawa	26 Aug 1934
11.6	Stanislawa Walasiewicz	POL	Berlin	1 Aug 1937
11.5	Fanny Blankers-Koen	NED	Amsterdam	13 Jun 1948
11.5	Marjorie Jackson	AUS	Helsinki	22 Jul 1952
11.4	Marjorie Jackson	AUS	Gifu	4 Oct 1952
11.3	Shirley Strickland	AUS	Warszawa	4 Aug 1955
11.3	Vera Krepkina	URS	Kiyev	13 Sep 1958
11.3	Wilma Rudolph	USA	Roma	2 Sep 1960
11.2	Wilma Rudolph	USA	Stuttgart	19 Jul 1961
11.2	Wyomia Tyus	USA	Tokyo	15 Oct 1964

100 Metres

Record	Name	Nationality	Venue	Date
11.1	Irena Kirszenstein	POL	Praha	9 Jul 1965
11.1	Wyomia Tyus	USA	Kiyev	31 Jul 1965
11.1	Barbara Ferrell	USA	Santa Barbara	2 Jul 1967
11.1	Lyudmila Samotyosova	URS	Leninakan	15 Aug 1968
11.1	Irena Kirzenstein/ Szewinska	POL	Ciudad de México	14 Oct 1968
11.0	Wyomia Tyus	USA	Ciudad de México	15 Oct 1968
11.0	Chi Cheng	TPE	Wien	18 Jul 1970
11.0	Renate Meissner	GDR	Berlin	2 Aug 1970
11.0	Renate Meissner/ Stecher	GDR	Berlin	31 Jul 1971
11.0	Renate Stecher	GDR	Potsdam	3 Jun 1972
11.0	Ellen Stropahl	GDR	Potsdam	15 Jun 1972
11.0	Eva Glesková	TCH	Budapest	1 Jul 1972
10.9	Renate Stecher	GDR	Ostrava	7 Jun 1973
10.8	Renate Stecher	GDR	Dresden	20 Jul 1973
Automatic timing:				
11.08	Wyomia Tyus	USA	Ciudad de México	15 Oct 1968
11.07	Renate Stecher	GDR	München	2 Sep 1972
11.04	Inge Helten	FRG	Fürth	13 Jun 1976
11.01	Annegret Richter	FRG	Montréal	25 Jul 1976
10.88	Marlies Oelsner	GDR	Dresden	1 Jul 1977
10.88	Marlies Oelsner/Göhr	GDR	Karl-Marx-Stadt	9 Jul 1982
10.81	Marlies Göhr	GDR	Berlin	8 Jun 1983
10.79	Evelyn Ashford	USA	USAF Academy	3 Jul 1983
10.76	Evelyn Ashford	USA	Zürich	22 Aug 1984
10.49	Florence Griffith Joyner	USA	Indianapolis	16 Jul 1988

(Note: Joyner's time above was probably strongly wind-assisted, and her 10.61 the following day should perhaps be regarded as the 'real' record.)

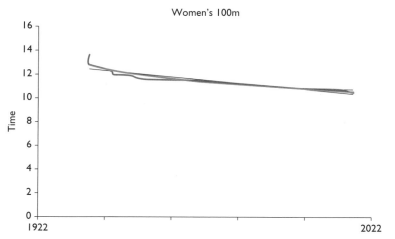

Women's 100m

Fig. 1.4: The progression of the IAAF World Record for the Women's 100m (blue line). The best-fit straight line is in black. The best-fit curve is in red. These predict the future.

200 Metres

y denotes 220 yards time equal to, or better than, the existing metric record

Record	Name	Nationality	Venue	Date
28.6	Marie Mejzlíková	TCH	Paris	21 May 1922
26.0	Eileen Edwards	GBR	Paris	3 Oct 1926
25.4	Eileen Edwards	GBR	Berlin	12 Jun 1927
24.7	Kinue Hitomi	JPN	Miyoshima	19 May 1929
24.6	Tollien Schuurman	NED	Bruxelles	13 Aug 1933
23.6	Stanislawa Walasiewicz	POL	Warszawa	4 Aug 1935
23.6	Marjorie Jackson	AUS	Helsinki	25 Jul 1952
23.4	Marjorie Jackson	AUS	Helsinki	25 Jul 1952
23.2	Betty Cuthbert	AUS	Sydney	16 Sep 1956
23.2y	Betty Cuthbert	AUS	Hobart	7 Mar 1960
22.9	Wilma Rudolph	USA	Corpus Christi	9 Jul 1960
22.9y	Margaret Burvill	AUS	Perth	22 Feb 1964
22.7	Irena Kirszenstein	POL	Warzawa	8 Aug 1965
22.5	Irena Kirszenstein/ Szewinska	POL	Ciudad de México	18 Oct 1968
22.4	Chi Cheng	TPE	München	12 Jul 1970
22.4	Renate Stecher	GDR	München	7 Sep 1972
22.1	Renate Stecher	GDR	Dresden	21 Jul 1973
Automatic timing:				
22.21	Irena Szewinska	POL	Potsdam	13 Jun 1974
22.06	Marita Koch	GDR	Erfurt	28 May 1978
22.02	Marita Koch	GDR	Leipzig	3 Jun 1979
21.71	Marita Koch	GDR	Karl-Marx-Stadt	10 Jun 1979

200 Metres

y denotes 220 yards time equal to, or better than, the existing metric record

Record	Name	Nationality	Venue	Date
21.71	Marita Koch	GDR	Potsdam	21 Jul 1984
21.71	Heike Drechsler	GDR	Jena	29 Jun 1986
21.71	Heike Drechsler	GDR	Stuttgart	29 Aug 1986
21.56	Florence Griffith Joyner	USA	Seoul	29 Sep 1988
21.34	Florence Griffith Joyner	USA	Seoul	29 Sep 1988

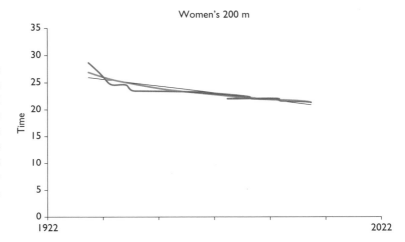

Women's 200 m

Fig. 1.5: The progression of the IAAF World Record for the Women's 200m (blue line). The best-fit straight line is in black. The best-fit curve is in red. These predict the future.

400 Metres

Records recognized by the IAAF from 1957, before which the best time on record was 53.9 by Mariya Itkina URS at Bucuresti on 1 Oct 1955.

y denotes 440 yards time equal to, or better than, the existing metric record

Record	Name	Nationality	Venue	Date
57.0y	Marlene Willard-Mathews	AUS	Sydney	6 Jan 1957
57.0y	Marise Chamberlain	NZL	Christchurch	16 Feb 1957
56.3y	Nancy Boyle	AUS	Sydney	24 Feb 1957
55.2	Polina Lazareva	URS	Moskva	10 May 1957
54.0	Mariya Itkina	URS	Minsk	8 Jun 1957
53.6	Mariya Itkina	URS	Moskva	6 Jul 1957
53.4	Mariya Itkina	URS	Krasnodar	12 Sep 1959
53.4	Mariya Itkina	URS	Beograd	14 Sep 1962
51.9	Shin Keum-dan	PRK	Pyongyang	23 Oct 1962
51.7	Nicole Duclos	FRA	Pireás	18 Sep 1969

400 Metres

Records recognized by the IAAF from 1957, before which the best time on record was 53.9 by Mariya Itkina URS at Bucuresti on 1 Oct 1955.

y denotes 440 yards time equal to, or better than, the existing metric record

Record	Name	Nationality	Venue	Date
51.7	Colette Besson	FRA	Pireás	18 Sep 1969
51.0	Marilyn Neufville	JAM	Edinburgh	23 Jul 1970
51.0	Monika Zehrt	GDR	Paris	4 Jul 1972
49.9	Irena Szewinska	POL	Warzawa	22 Jun 1974
Automatic timing:				
50.14	Riitta Salin	FIN	Roma	4 Sep 1974
49.77	Christina Brehmer	GDR	Dresden	9 May 1976
49.75	Irena Szewinska	POL	Bydgoszcz	22 Jun 1976
49.29	Irena Szewinska	POL	Montréal	29 Jul 1976
49.19	Marita Koch	GDR	Leipzig	2 Jul 1978
49.03	Marita Koch	GDR	Potsdam	19 Aug 1978
48.94	Marita Koch	GDR	Praha	31 Aug 1978
48.89	Marita Koch	GDR	Potsdam	29 Jul 1979
48.60	Marita Koch	GDR	Torino	4 Aug 1979
48.16	Marita Koch	GDR	Athína	8 Sep 1982
47.99	Jarmila Kratochvílová	TCH	Helsinki	10 Aug 1983
47.60	Marita Koch	GDR	Canberra	6 Oct 1985

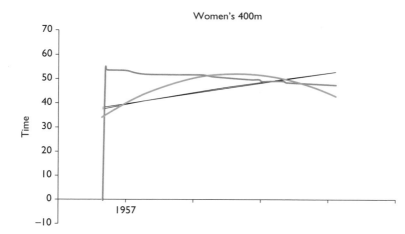

Fig. 1.6: The progression of the IAAF World Record for the Women's 400m (blue line). The best-fit straight line is in black. The best-fit curve is in red. These predict the future.

CHAPTER 2

TALENT IDENTIFICATION AND DEVELOPMENT IN SPRINTING

by Dr Mohsen Shafizadeh

So, is 'talent' a myth or a reality? This is an important question that has been posed for many decades across different aspects of life, such as business and sport. Many efforts have been made to ensure that the recruitment of human resources in any profession is carried out according to an approved, scientific framework, rather than by simple chance.

In sport we hear a lot about successful athletes who repeatedly break world records and dominate their sport for long periods: talented Olympic and World Champions such as Usain Bolt in sprinting, who has won fourteen gold medals; Sir Steven Redgrave in rowing, who won fourteen gold medals; Naim Süleymanoğlu in weightlifting, who won ten gold medals; Roger Federer in tennis, who has won seventeen grand slam singles titles; Tiger Woods in golf, who has won fourteen majors; and Lionel Messi in association football, who was voted Player of the Year for three successive years – and there are many others who have excelled in sport and brought new horizons to the former perceived limitations of human performance.

Talking about athletes, and the talents they possess, has long been a challenging topic, and has drawn together a wide range of scientists to debate the parameters that predict successful performance. Geneticists have attempted to define talented athletes through their innate abilities and capacities, which are defined by heredity. On the other hand, coaches and practitioners have been interested in associating talent development with environmental factors, and specifically the effects of practice.

The debate between nature and nurture – or between genetics and environment – has long been a source of discussion in education and psychology, and, more recently, in sports science and sports coaching. Regardless of the ways in which a successful performance is generated, what is interesting is the way that we define our expectations of an athlete in the coaching process. This introduces different models of talent identification and development in sport, which have been used in many countries.

The human physical domain has a range of functions. 'Speed' and 'ability to react' are two of the key physical components that have been identified as basic motor abilities and requirements for many sports (Schorer & Elfeink-Gemser, 2013). The key questions for coaches who work with sprinters are how to identify gifted athletes, and whether it is possible to increase their limits beyond pre-determined capacities.

This chapter will attempt to employ the latest sports science to answer these questions, the first part generically, and the second part in relation to sprint events specifically. After this, important elements in sprinting are discussed in more detail, and finally the models of prediction and talent development are explained in full.

NATURE VERSUS NURTURE

The record of Caribbean athletes in the history of sprinting is outstanding and amazing. The athletes from Jamaica, Trinidad-and-Tobago, Bahamas and Barbados, together with Caribbean migrants now residing in countries such as the USA, Canada and Great Britain, have shone in recent decades at Olympic Games and World Championships.

In fact it is not easy to explain the outstanding success of black athletes purely by reference to their race *per se*, and there is a dilemma between genetics and environment in shaping talented sprinters. Jamaican athletes have won many medals recently, and at the top of the list is Usain Bolt with his fourteen gold medals. Which factors differentiate Caribbean sprinters from those who originate from other parts of the planet?

The answer might be in the story of a biologist who spent many years in Africa and Jamaica distinguishing between the facts and the myths of successful performance in sprint events (Epstein, 2014). Yannis Pitsiladis from Glasgow University is a professor in genetics who has worked in sport science for the

last decade. He was interested in knowing whether genetics played an important role in the development of gifted sprinters from Jamaica. He interviewed different groups of people and sampled their DNA for analysis in his laboratory.

When he asked Jamaican people about their superiority in sprinting, many of them had differing ideas. Some attributed their success to the use of specific yams, some to the habit of young people running everywhere, and some to the need to escape from European slave masters. He found that the most gifted sprinters, such as Usain Bolt and Veronica Campbell-Brown, had been nurtured in a specific part of the island: Trelawney.

The 'escape of slaves' story does not seem unrealistic in the forming of future champions in a small part of the planet. In fact, slaves were warriors who had to fight and invade other countries on the orders of their masters. Many of them came from West Africa, from countries such as Ghana, Nigeria, Cameroon and Gabon. Maroon's fighters have spread out and created a history in sprint events. Genetic studies of Jamaican ancestry have found an array of West African lineage. For example, the Y-chromosome of Jamaicans tended to be most similar to that of Africans from the Bight of Biafra. In fact, the genetic pattern of Jamaicans is very similar to that of West Africans, but from different countries. On the other hand, because of Spanish colonizers, some communities in Jamaica, such as the Taino, have DNA from white people from America.

Pitsiladis' study also showed that Jamaicans are very diverse when it comes to the ACT3 (sprint) gene. Nearly all Jamaicans have a copy of the best version of the gene for sprinting. Generally, Pitsiladis' theory regarding the role of genetic variation in Jamaican sprinters has been influenced less by the data he has compiled with extensive DNA sequences and chromatography. So, maybe other factors are important in creating the world's best sprint factory in this island, rather than just genetics.

'Champs' is a recognized national high school competition that has taken place in Jamaica since 1910. It is an event that demonstrates the abilities of young Jamaican sprinters to the world. Many young people take part in this event in order to secure scholarships available to athletes in American colleges. The Jamaican sprint system is similar to the United States system in football. In fact, many coaches give household items such as refrigerators to parents in order to recruit their children.

Some of the great Jamaican sprinters were originally interested in other sports. For example, Usain Bolt's first choice was cricket, and then soccer. His close training partner, Yohan Blake, wanted to be a cricketer. However, both were encouraged to select track-and-field over their original preferences as a result of their performances in Champs competitions. The sprint results at Champs are actually comparable to those at state championship meets in big sprinting states such as Texas. In the Jamaican system, nearly every child is compelled to sprint in youth races at some point. They develop their performance very slowly, but Champs gives them a great opportunity to perform on a big stage and see the opportunities for a better life.

How much practice is necessary in order to improve performance? What is the impact of deliberate practice on the development of sport expertise? What do we know about the triangular interaction of motivation, readiness and learning on a successful performance? These are questions that reveal the superiority of talented athletes in sport.

The influential role of practice on performance and motor skills has been proposed since the 1800s through a work by Bryan and Harter on the telegrapher's skill. They suggested that the accumulation of effort and practice over time can enhance skill proficiency. Their suggestion was known as the 'power law of practice', in which the learning progress in the early part of practice is significant but gradually decreases as practice continues. Later, scientists were interested to understand how much practice is necessary to create an expert in different professions.

Studies of chess players by Simon and Chase, later replicated by Ericsson on athletes from other sports, revealed the importance of ten years – or 10,000 hours practice – in achieving expertise in an activity (Baker and Cobley, 2013). Ericsson (1993) suggested that the only way to develop expertise in sport, or any profession, is by following the deliberate practice principle in which an athlete has to complete 10,000 hours of commitment and purposeful effort on a specific activity. The deliberate practice model of expertise holds that talent does not exist, or makes a negligible contribution to performance, and that initial performance will be unrelated to achieving expertise, and that ten years of deliberate practice is necessary.

Sprint events are largely determined by the function of muscle fibres. Everyone is born with a mixture of the three types of muscle fibre: Type I (also known as slow-twitch), Type IIa (intermediate fast-twitch) and Type IIb (super-fast-twitch). Fast-twitch fibres are characterized by a fast speed of contraction and relaxation, high force capacity and a low threshold for fatigue (McArdle, Katch and Katch, 1996). Because of the nature of sprinting, sprinters possess a high percentage of fast-twitch fibres. It is estimated that sprinters who run in 100–200m events have 65 per cent fast-twitch muscle fibres (Bergh et al., 1977).

How much the make-up of muscle fibre is determined by genetic factors, and how much it is determined by training or activity, is subject to considerable controversy in the scientific community. While most people acknowledge that fibres can be converted within type (that is, from Type IIa to Type IIb or vice versa), many argue that there is no simple way to truly convert from one type to another.

A study by Lombardo and Deaner, 2014, looked at the performance of sprinters before formal training to see whether the model applied, and found that in almost every case, world-class sprinters were exceptional before they started training. The findings showed that firstly, a strong predictor, probably a pre-condition, for elite sprinting performance is exceptional speed prior to formal training; secondly, that this exceptional ability is at least partly specific to sprinting; and thirdly, that many elite sprinters reach world-class status in far less than ten years, although they usually make modest improvements even after that.

If sprinters are born rather than made, and if the ten-year rule is not applicable to sprint events, then the role of practice on sprint performance might be beyond physiological limits and more towards mechanical changes in technique and movement patterns. Deshon and Nelson (see Hay, 1993) found a significant positive correlation between the angle the leg made with the ground at the instant the foot landed, and the speed of running.

The agonistic and antagonistic muscles also become better coordinated, in that the antagonists furnish less resistance to the contractile efforts of the agonists. The speed of a sprinter is a product of stride length and stride frequency, and every sprinter has to determine the best balance between those two factors, depending on his or her size. The runner must continue to fully extend his or her stride without over-striding, where the optimum placing of the feet with each stride is at a point in relation to his or her body, where the centre of gravity remains exactly midway between the feet. These elements are improved through practice because they are skill-based factors of sprint events.

THE INGREDIENTS OF TALENTED ATHLETES

One way to categorize sport performance is by employing the notion of ability-skill diversity in individual performers. In fact, the necessity to understand the needs of a particular sport through task analysis would be a good guideline for practitioners to design appropriate training environments. The general idea regarding the diversity of human performance in any discipline is based on the individual difference principle. Every athlete is unique because each possesses an individual set of motor abilities and varying proficiency in motor skills. In fact, the quality of performance depends on how we use different abilities to create a skill or technique.

It should be stressed that abilities and skills are two different concepts, and that the former is a prerequisite for the latter. Motor abilities are defined as genetically determined traits that are stable and enduring, and which underlie the execution of sport skills. In terms of number and commonality, they are relatively few and exist in all people. It is believed that motor abilities, because they are genetically defined, are unchanged by practice or environmental conditions (Edwards, 2011). Motor skills, on the other hand, are defined as acquired, changeable and modified by practice and experience, and as not necessarily existing equally in all people.

Skills depend on ability, are observable, and vary over time (Schmidt and Wrisberg, 2011). Because there are a fixed number of motor abilities, any superiority in sporting performance may be directly related to the strength and balance of those abilities. For example, we all possess fast- and slow-twitch fibres, but the main difference between sprinters and distance runners is the distribution of fast- and slow-twitch fibres in the target muscles. As mentioned above, it is estimated that sprinters who run in 100–200m events have 65 per cent fast-twitch muscle fibres (Bergh *et al.*, 1978) – that is, 10 to 15 per cent more than in the average population.

Understanding the difference between motor abilities and skills for talent identification and development is of paramount importance, but the critical question for coaches who work with athletes is how to identify the determined abilities. In order to answer this question, the Fleishman taxonomy of motor abilities (Fleishman, 1972) is very informative. Fleishman classified motor abilities into perceptual motor and physical proficiency categories that are different in terms of involvement of the nervous system and physiological factors.

The perceptual motor abilities are comprised of those motor abilities in which the central nervous system is the primary determinant of the ability's relative strength, whereas physical proficiency motor abilities depend upon physiological factors such as body composition, the mechanical properties of the muscles and the proficiency of receptors in addition to the nervous system. The table shows the definition of different motor abilities according to Fleishman's taxonomy.

After identification of associated motor abilities for a particular sport skill (for example, sprinting) the next task for practitioners and coaches is to determine the amount of the contribution. For example, how much multi-limb coordination is required for the successful performance of sprinting events (0–100 per cent)? This kind of task analysis is very useful in terms of identifying underling motor abilities in the prediction of successful performance. For example, two

children who differ on response orientation as an important ability in sprint events will demonstrate different levels of trainability in the start phase of the race. For coaches who work with these children, it is essential to design appropriate, individualized, training programmes to enhance their potential.

PREDICTION OF EXPERT PERFORMANCE

One of the problems in talent development is the prediction of successful performance, or the time to attain expert performance. Due to the variety of physical and physiological capacities and the maturation of different body systems, the time taken to respond to any organized training programme varies (Malina, Bouchard, Bar-Or, 2004). On the other hand, prediction of trainability according to information from screening tests in the early phase of talent identification is not always successful and robust (Schmidt and Wrisberg, 2011).

One reason behind this fact is the change in the pattern of underlying abilities over time. For example, if abilities A, B and C are determinants of successful performance at novice level, their contribution because of practice and experience is changed at expert level. According to Ackerman's model, the importance of cognitive, perceptual motor and physical abilities in the process of motor learning is different, because of their role in the prediction of performance (Ackerman, 1992).

For a novice sprinter in early training, the most important elements to acquire are the ability to understand the mechanics of movement pattern, and using memory to store information. Gradually, he/she needs to strengthen perceptual and speed abilities in

FLEISHMAN'S TAXONOMY OF MOTOR ABILITIES
(FLEISHMAN *ET AL.*, 1984)

Perceptual motor abilities

Multi-limb coordination   Ability to coordinate the movement of a number of limbs simultaneously. A high level of this ability is probably important for running, skipping and hopping

Control precision   Ability to make highly controlled movement adjustments, particularly when large muscle groups are involved. This ability is important for hurdle sprint events that require careful positioning of the feet

Response orientation   Ability to make quick choices among numerous alternative actions, often measured as choice reaction time. Start position in sprint events requires response to a specific stimulus

Rate control   Ability to produce continuous anticipatory movement adjustments in response to changes in the speed of a moving target. Example includes auto racing

Manual dexterity   Ability to manipulate relatively large objects with the hands and arms. An example is shot putt throwing

Finger dexterity   Ability to manipulate small objects. An example is dart throwing

Arm–hand steadiness   Ability to make precise arm and hand positioning movements where strength and speed are not required. An example is holding a gun for shooting

Wrist–finger speed   Ability to rapidly move the wrist and fingers with little or no accuracy demands. An example is typing

Aiming   Ability that requires the production of accurate hand movements to targets under speed conditions. An example is rapidly hitting a target

Physical proficiency abilities

Explosive strength   Ability to expend a maximum of energy in one explosive act. Examples of tasks requiring this ability include jumping, throwing and 100m race

Static strength   Ability to exert force against a relatively heavy weight or some immovable object. Task requiring high levels of static strength include weight lifting

Dynamic strength   Ability to repeatedly or continuously move or support the weight of the body such as rope climbing and ring performance in gymnastics

Trunk strength   Dynamic strength that is particular to the trunk and abdominal muscles. An example is pommel horse in gymnastics

Extent flexibility   Ability to extend and stretch the body as far as possible in various directions. An example is yoga

Dynamic flexibility   Ability to make repeated, rapid movements requiring muscle flexibility. An example is hurdle sprint race

Gross body equilibrium   Ability to maintain total body balance in the absence of vision

Balance   Ability to maintain total body balance with vision. An example is performance on the balance beam

Speed of limb   Ability to move the arms or legs quickly, but without reaction time stimulus, to minimize movement time. This ability is important in sprint events

Gross body coordination   Ability to perform a number of complex movements simultaneously. An example is circus performance

Stamina   Ability to exert the entire body for a prolonged period of time, such as distance running

Abilities that are associated with sprint events are highlighted in *italic* order to respond to environmental stimuli. Finally, the sprinter requires motor abilities such as multi-limb coordination, explosive strength and flexibility in the expert level of skill acquisition.

The attainment of expert performance requires high-level commitment and spending ten years of deliberate practice. According to Bloom's model (1985) there are three phases of expert development in sport. The first phase begins with an individual's introduction to activities in a particular sport, and ends with the start of instruction and deliberate practice. The second phase consists of an extended period of preparation, and ends with the individual's commitment to pursue activities in the sport on a full-time basis. The third phase consists of full-time commitment to improving performance, and ends when the individual either can make a living as professional performer, or terminates full-time engagement in the sport.

Athletes dropping out have always been an issue in youth sport. Even innate ability and potential are not always enough to overcome injury, lack of motivation, alternative interests and other personal and environmental factors (Payne and Issacs, 2012). Talented athletes face a range of constraints capable of limiting their ability to achieve exceptional levels of performance. These constraints usually relate to resources, effort and motivation.

RESOURCE CONSTRAINTS (ERICSSON, *ET AL.*, 1993)

The history of sport is littered with talented athletes who failed to achieve their potential due to a lack of access to resources. According to interviews with international-level performers, their first exposure to deliberate practice was usually between the ages of three and eight. At this age, the only transport facilities available to children to sport facilities are parents and guardians. The other barriers to participation are access to facilities and financial support. Parents are frequently required to devote considerable amounts of time and money to deliver their children to training and competition, and sometimes have to contemplate moving their home closer to the facilities.

When travel and accommodation costs are added to the purchase of essential kit and of necessary supplements, then it is not impossible that the costs of participation exceed the family income.

At each stage of an athlete's development, consideration must be given to the costs involved, the motivation of the athlete and the results being achieved, with the final stages of development being the most expensive (Bloom, 1985).

EFFORT CONSTRAINTS

The degree of physical and mental effort necessary to develop a consistently high performer in sport is of paramount importance. Sustaining deliberate practice for an extended period of months and years requires a balance of exertion and rest. It has been estimated that twice as many athletes overtrain as undertrain. Elite sprinting requires great strength and speed, and training that consists of short-burst activity so that longer periods of recovery are recommended (McArdle, Katch and Katch, 1996).

Research has shown that when performing high-quality sprint training, it is best to limit the duration of training to just two hours: a balance of quality and quantity (Welford, 1968). Coaches need to review not only the amount of sprint training, but the amount of strength training, conditioning and so on, as well as the physiological and psychological stresses that their charges are experiencing.

Another limiting factor to achieving high-level performances is the risk of injury to runners. Frequent exposure to maximum effort, combined with insufficient opportunities for recovery between sessions, will increase the chance of shin splints and Achilles tendonitis (Subotnick, 1977) as well as gradually causing staleness, overtraining and, eventually, burnout.

The duration of practice is very limited in the early phases of deliberate practice. Most international performers start with a short duration (10–20min) of long-term training programmes (Bloom, 1985). Consistent with the idea of slow adaptation to the demands of extended practice, individuals are encouraged to adopt a regular weekly schedule with relatively fixed duration. The increase in the amount of practice should be gradual and slow to avoid the risk of overtraining (Hackney, Pearman, and Novack, 1990).

MOTIVATIONAL CONSTRAINTS

Motivating children and talented young athletes to sustain their efforts over the long term requires close communication between the athlete, the parents and the coaches. Children have to feel comfortable and enjoy their activities in order to sustain their deliberate practice for an extended period of time. According to Bloom (1985), parents generally delay for several months before agreeing to support their children in deliberate practice, preferring to observe their children engaged in playful practice and expressing their interest in deliberate practice before committing the time and money that this requires.

This social support from parents and others is very important in establishing the initial motivation. Gradually, children can build up the internal motivation with the support of coaches and instructors, and with increased experience. As performers become more involved in a particular sport, competitions provide short-term goals for specific improvements. At this stage, the motivation to practise is closely connected to the goal of becoming an expert performer, and will be an integral part of fast- and slow-twitch fibres in the individual's daily life.

If individuals enjoy deliberate practice, they ought to practise at a uniformly high level all year. On the other hand, many athletes who have practised for a long period of time give up their aspirations to compete and excel in an activity. Without the ambition to improve performance, the motivation to engage in the activity is reduced or vanishes.

In summary, the prediction of expert performance through the amount of deliberate practice depends on two factors. Firstly, the past amount of deliberate practice is directly related to the individual's current performance, while expert performance is not reached with less than sufficient years (meaning the ten-year rule, or 10,000 hours in most sports) of deliberate practice. Secondly, deliberate practice starts at low levels and increases slowly over time.

CHAPTER 3

BIOMECHANICAL ANALYSIS OF THE TECHNIQUES OF THE SPRINT START

by Professor Morteza Shahbazi Moghaddam

Sprinting is the act of running over a short distance at (or near) top speed. It is used in many sports that incorporate running, typically as a way of quickly reaching a target or goal, or catching or avoiding an opponent. Human physiology dictates that a sprinter cannot maintain top speed (or even close to it) for more than 30–35 seconds, due to the accumulation of lactic acid in the muscles.

Sprinting involves a quick-acceleration phase followed by a speed-maintenance phase. During the initial stages of sprinting, as the runner drives out of the starting blocks, they tilt their upper body forwards in order to direct ground reaction forces more horizontally. As they reach their maximum velocity, the torso straightens out into an upright position.

The goal of sprinting is to reach and maintain a high top speed in order to cover a set distance in the shortest possible time. A lot of research has been invested in quantifying the biological factors and the mathematics and mechanics that govern sprinting. In order to achieve these high velocities, it has been found that sprinters have to apply a considerable amount of force on to the ground in order to achieve the desired acceleration, rather than taking more rapid steps.

Biomechanics is a type of engineering, as it often uses traditional engineering sciences to analyse human movement. Although simple applications of Newtonian mechanics and materials sciences can provide reasonable approximations to the mechanics of the human body, it is applied mechanics – most notably mechanical engineering disciplines such as structural analysis, kinematics, kinetics and dynamics – that plays the more prominent role in the study of biomechanics. On the other hand, since the human body is a complex system, numerical methods are notably applied in almost every biomechanical study.

In sports biomechanics, the laws of mechanics are applied to human movement in order to gain a greater understanding of athletic performance, and to reduce the incidence of sports injury. In order to achieve all biomechanical parameters during the execution of a given task by the athlete, many tools have been developed to assist in the assessment of running gait. These include the more traditional motion capture systems used to describe the motion of the body, force plates that quantify the forces acting on the body, and electromyography (EMG) used to estimate the level of muscle activity during motion.

More recently, smaller, portable sensors have been developed, which may be used successfully to measure the parameters of gait. These include accelerometers, electro-goniometers, gyroscopes, and in-sole pressure sensors (see box). These tools have been successfully used to investigate shoe, orthotic performance, risk factors for injury, running performance, fatigue effects, and gait adaptations to various running techniques.

THE SPRINT START

Block Start Phase

In any sprinting, the start is the most important factor in predicting success. Starting blocks have been used in track races up to 400m under International Association of Athletic Federations (IAAF) rules since the London Olympics of 1948. The block start phase refers to the period that the sprinter is in contact with the blocks. Sprinters take comfort in the psychological feel-good factor of the starting block distance between the posterior and the front, but discomfort in the physiological discord between the soleus and the gastrocnemius. The crouch start commences from a position where both feet and both hands are in contact with the ground.

The key to success is finding a method of starting that best suits the athlete concerned, taking into account physique, ability, experience and strength. There are basically three different types of crouch start technique: the bunch or bullet start (<30cm), the elongated start (>50cm), and the medium start (30–50cm); most sprinters and hurdlers employ a technique that is somewhere between two of these.

Velocity is proportional to the product of force and time. In other words velocity, particularly from the crouch start, is produced by exerting a strong force for a long period of time. In the start, therefore, the legs must be in the best anatomical position to produce the greatest possible force for the longest practicable time.

The bullet start can produce a great force but only for a very short period of time. The elongated start permits force to be exerted for a longer period but restricts the amount of force generated, particularly by the rear leg. The medium start is a compromise between the fast clearance produced by the bullet start, and the extended duration of the elongated start.

The block start phase begins when the starter gives the command 'On your marks', continues through his command 'Set' and the firing of the gun, and ends when the athlete leaves the blocks (see Fig. 3.1).

On hearing the command 'On your marks', the athlete steps up to the start and adopts a position with the hands shoulder-width apart and just behind the starting line. The feet are in contact with the starting blocks and the knee of the rear leg is in contact with the track.

On the command 'Set', the athlete straightens the rear leg so as to raise the knee off the ground and thereby elevate the hip and shift the body's centre of mass (CM) up and out. When the gun is fired the athlete reacts by driving both legs against the blocks and into the first running strides (see Fig. 3.1(a) to (h)).

SENSORS USED TO MEASURE THE PARAMETERS OF GAIT

The following are some of the sensors very commonly used to measure the parameters of gait.

Electromyography

Electromyography (EMG) is a technique commonly used to measure the levels of muscle activity during the walking or running gait. Typically, the timing of muscle activation and its relative intensity are the primary measures of interest and can be collected through the use of surface or indwelling (fine-wire) electrodes. This technique can be used to detect abnormal gait behaviour and to assess the neuromuscular control of a runner.

Motion analysis

The most common method for collecting information about the position and orientation of body segments in two- or three-dimensional space is the use of motion capture technology (often referred to as 'stereophotogrammetry'), in which markers are affixed to the subject and tracked throughout the motion of interest.

Force plates

Force plates are commonly used to measure contact forces between the foot and the ground (ground reaction force – GRF). This information can be used to quantify impact forces, loading rates, as well as propulsive and breaking forces, and to track changes in the centre of pressure over time.

Pressure sensors

The use of in-shoe pressure sensors provides a lightweight, portable and easy-to-use alternative by which to analyse running gait. Unlike force platforms, they are capable of quantifying the distribution of force over the plantar surface of the foot, providing more detailed information on the loading of the foot during gait than force measures alone. Because this device is placed in the shoe, the loads acting on the foot surface can be measured directly, as opposed to the force acting on the bottom of the shoe with a standard force platform.

Accelerometers

The use of body-fixed sensors such as accelerometers is rapidly becoming a viable alternative to more traditional gait analysis techniques in the assessment of human motion. Accelerometers are inertial sensors that provide a direct measurement of acceleration along single or multiple axes, effectively reducing the error associated with the differentiation of displacement and velocity data derived from sources such as motion capture systems.

Electrogoniometers

Electrogoniometers allow the direct measurement of joint angles during continuous dynamic activities. They offer a simple, affordable alternative to motion capture systems and allow joint-angle data to be collected and viewed instantaneously. The end blocks of the electrogoniometers are typically affixed to the skin on either side of the joint axis of rotation using double-sided adhesive tape, as specified by the manufacturer.

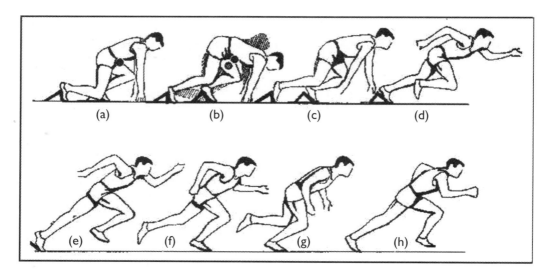

Fig. 3.1: Adapted from J. G. Hay *The Biomechanics of Sports Techniques* **3rd edition 1983: (a) 'On your marks'; (b) 'Set'; (c) 'Go'; (d) block release; (e) rear leg extension and the first step of flight; (f) right leg landing; (g) preparation of the second step; (h) right leg extension.**

As the athlete straightens up, the hands are no longer in contact with the track, and he or she can start to swing the arms vigorously.

The purpose of the block start is to facilitate a fast and effective start to the race. The main objectives of the athlete during this phase can be summarized as follows:

- To establish a balanced position on the blocks
- To obtain a body position with the CM as high as is practical and slightly forward of the base of support
- To apply a force against the blocks whose line of action goes through the ankle, knee and hip joints, the centre of the trunk and the head
- To apply this force against the blocks and through the body at an angle of approximately 45 degrees
- To clear the blocks with the greatest possible velocity and acceleration

START STATIC DESCRIPTION

To better understand the biomechanics of the sprint start, four distinct phases, with precise beginning and end points, are detailed below.

Phase I: The 'on your marks' position, in which the major joint contributions come from the shoulders, which have to support the weight of the upper body *and* withstand the drive from the legs against the hands. This phase starts when the feet and hands are placed, and the knees are touching the ground, and ends when the body becomes motionless, waiting for the 'set' command.

Phase II: The 'set' position, which uses the hips, knees and shoulders. The hips and knees thrust the pelvis upwards, while the hands and arms support the upper body. This phase begins when the knees and hips are thrust upwards on the 'set' command, and ends when the body becomes motionless awaiting the gun.

Phase III: The 'go' position, where the rear leg drives 'explosively' out of the blocks, with the hip, knee and ankle extending fully and dynamically. This phase begins when the body starts accelerating in a linear motion on the 'go' signal, and ends when the rear foot leaves the blocks.

Phase IV: 'First step (release)/front leg extension'. This final phase utilizes the hip, knee and ankle of the front leg, and the lower back to pull the body upwards. The shoulders and arms are now only supporting the arms' weight as well as all inertia created by the motion. The beginning of the phase is when the rear leg and front arm are in a forward motion; the phase ends when the front leg is fully extended and rear arm is extended above the body figure (see Fig. 3.2).

Block Spacing

Much of the early research on the sprint start focused on the effects of adjusting the position of the blocks in an attempt to manipulate 'set' position kinematics experimentally. It is widely accepted that increasing the distance between the two blocks induces an increase in total block force and in push duration, and thus greater total block impulses and hence block velocities. Whilst the front foot forces have been found to be independent of inter-block spacing, more elongated starts lead to greater forces being exerted by the rear foot. However, whether these increases actually represent an improvement in performance is less clear.

As stated previously, the choice of performance measure with which to assess the effects of such an intervention can influence

its perceived success. Research has shown that a relative time loss is incurred when generating a forceful push against the blocks. This had led to the widespread acceptance that an intermediate interblock spacing provides the best platform for block phase performance, allowing sprinters to generate relatively large forces without spending detrimental amounts of time doing so.

It is also suggested that positioning the CM ('centre of mass') as close to the start line as possible is important in sprinting, as it moves the sprinter closer to the finish line, thus reducing the total distance to be covered during a race. This is achieved not only by reducing the interblock distance, but also by reducing the distance between the front block and the start line. When adjusting this distance, it has been found that there is a small but statistically non-significant decrease in the time taken to reach 10m as the distance between the front block and the start line is reduced. Reis and Fazenda (2004) measured the distance between the front block and the start line as chosen by fifteen male sprinters (of unstated ability level).

The authors found a moderately strong, significant relationship between this distance and the time taken to reach 20m and 60m, suggesting that those sprinters who reached these distances earlier adopted a front-foot position closer to the start line. However, the causality of this cannot be determined, and it may relate to the suggestions that the faster sprinters are able to adopt such positions in the blocks due to their greater strength.

Initial Steps of a Sprint

As highlighted above, the choice of either block velocity or the time taken to reach 10m as a performance measure can be considered as two important keys in the sprint start. This

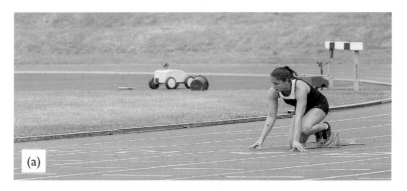

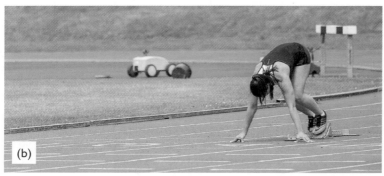

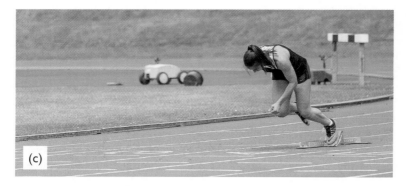

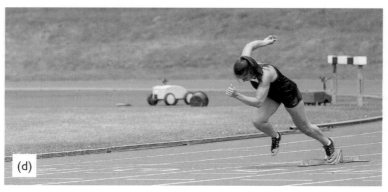

Fig. 3.2 (a–g):
Successive photos
illustrating (a) 'On
your marks', (b) 'Go',
(c) 'Release', and the
first and second steps
(d) to (g), where the
trunk is still bent.
(Photos: Darren
Charles Holloway)

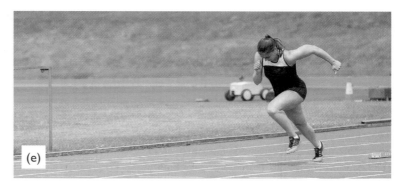

Fig. 3.2 (*continued*)

(e)

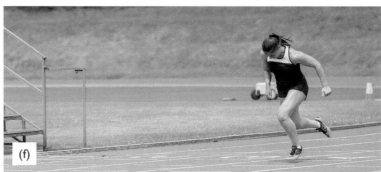

(f)

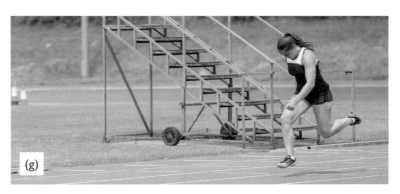

(g)

implies that adjustments can be made by a sprinter during the early steps of a sprint in order to reduce the time taken to cover a specific distance despite a lower block velocity. The initial post-block steps during a sprint start thus possess the potential to have a considerable effect upon the performance. Sprinters continue to accelerate rapidly after leaving the blocks as they strive to achieve their maximum velocity.

This acceleration is an important part of a sprint, because if a sprinter is able to reach his/her maximum velocity earlier, the time spent running at sub-maximal velocities will be reduced, thus reducing the time taken to cover a specific sprint distance. Numerous biomechanical investigations have so far been undertaken on the block phase regarding the technique of sprinters during the initial steps after block exit.

Block Obliquity

One further feature of the block settings which can be manipulated by the sprinter is the angle of the block faces. Several researchers have therefore conducted studies where these block obliquities have been altered experimentally, and the consequent effects on performance determined. Guissard et al. (1992) found that as front block obliquity decreased from 70 to 50 degrees and then 30 degrees (relative to the track), start parameters such as mean block velocity increased from 2.37, 2.80 and 2.94m/sec respectively, and block acceleration increased from 7.46, 8.36 and 9.03m/sec² respectively without affecting the total duration of the push phase.

The authors suggested that the improvement in start performance with decreasing block obliquity could be attributed to an increased contribution by the medial gastrocnemius muscle during the eccentric and concentric phases of calf muscle contraction, due to an earlier onset. This increased contraction was deemed to be a result of progressive lengthening of the soleus and gastrocnemius muscles in the 'Set' position as the front block obliquity decreased. Cousins and Dyson (2004) altered the obliquities of both blocks independently, and recorded the forces produced against each block by five sprinters of unstated ability level.

It was found that the greatest horizontal forces were achieved using the smallest angles at each block (30 degrees on the front block, 50 degrees on the rear). Mero et al. (2006) also altered the angle of both block faces (either both at 40 degrees or both at 65 degrees), and calculated joint kinetics and muscle-tendon lengths throughout the block phase. The results again revealed that smaller block angles induced greater block velocities. Mero et al. (2006) determined that these increased block velocities were largely due to elongated initial muscle-tendon lengths of the gastrocnemius and soleus, which contributed to greater peak ankle moments and powers, and thus higher block velocities, confirming the previous theories of Guissard et al. (1992).

Joints and Muscles Involved

The main joints involved in the start position are shoulder, trunk, knee and ankle. While the shoulder joint is mainly used for equilibrium, especially in the set position, the trunk, knee and ankle joints are used to propel the athlete to release the start block with as high an acceleration as possible. The muscles involved are mainly the erector spinae, gluteus maximus, rectus femoris, vastus medialis, vastus lateralis, biceps femoris and gastrocnemius, which are used to propel the athlete from the starting blocks, while the shoulder muscles such as deltoid, subscapularis and infraspinatus are used to provide athlete equilibrium in the 'set' position. A typical raw electromyographs of selected muscles in the front and rear legs during a maximal block start of a typical subject is shown in Fig. 3.4, in which the ground reaction force (horizontal and vertical components) and total reaction time are also shown (from Mero and Komi, 1990).

MUSCLE ACTIVITY

Electromyography (EMG) is currently used in athlete performance to record muscle activity during the sprint start. The gluteus maximus of the rear leg has been observed to be the first muscle active during the block phase (Mero and Komi, 1990; Čoh et al., 2007), whilst Guissard and Duchateau (1990) observed the biceps femoris to be the first muscle recruited in both legs, although they did not collect data from the gluteus maximus.

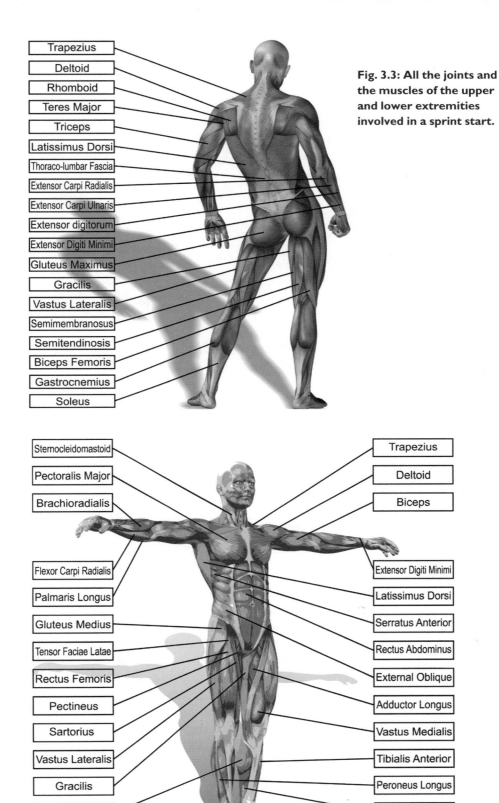

Fig. 3.3: All the joints and the muscles of the upper and lower extremities involved in a sprint start.

Trapezius
Deltoid
Rhomboid
Teres Major
Triceps
Latissimus Dorsi
Thoraco-lumbar Fascia
Extensor Carpi Radialis
Extensor Carpi Ulnaris
Extensor digitorum
Extensor Digiti Minimi
Gluteus Maximus
Gracilis
Vastus Lateralis
Semimembranosus
Semitendinosis
Biceps Femoris
Gastrocnemius
Soleus

Sternocleidomastoid
Pectoralis Major
Brachioradialis
Flexor Carpi Radialis
Palmaris Longus
Gluteus Medius
Tensor Faciae Latae
Rectus Femoris
Pectineus
Sartorius
Vastus Lateralis
Gracilis
Gastrocnemius
Extensor Digitorum Brevis

Trapezius
Deltoid
Biceps
Extensor Digiti Minimi
Latissimus Dorsi
Serratus Anterior
Rectus Abdominus
External Oblique
Adductor Longus
Vastus Medialis
Tibialis Anterior
Peroneus Longus
Soleus
Extensor Hallucis Brevis

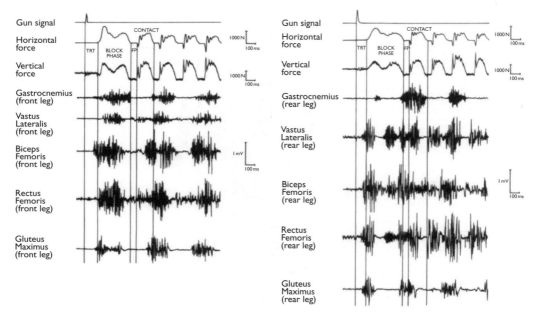

Fig. 3.4: Raw electromyographs of selected muscles in the front and rear legs during a maximal block start of one subject. TRT = total reaction time; FP = flight phase. The ground reaction force (horizontal and vertical components) is also displayed (adopted from Mero and Komi, 1990).

Rear leg biceps femoris activation is found to be followed shortly after by quadriceps (rectus femoris, vastus lateralis and vastus medialis) and then calf muscle (soleus and gastrocnemius) activation (Guissard and Duchateau, 1990): see Fig. 3.5.

The rear leg quadriceps have been found to be typically only active during the early part of the rear block push phase, deactivating prior to the rear foot leaving the block to keep this foot clear of the track during the subsequent rear leg swing phase (Guissard and Duchateau, 1990; Čoh et al., 2007). During the remainder of rear block contact, only the biceps femoris and calf muscles were found to remain active (Guissard and Duchateau, 1990).

In the front leg, the vastii muscles have been typically found to be active throughout virtually the entire drive phase in the

blocks, activating soon after the initial gluteus maximus and biceps femoris activation, and remaining active almost until the instant of block exit (Fig. 3.5). In contrast to the vastii muscles of the quadriceps, the rectus femoris muscle only becomes active during the late part of the block phase, potentially due to its biarticular nature being a limiter of early hip extension.

The front leg soleus has been observed to activate considerably earlier than the gastrocnemius muscle, which was suggested to be due to knee flexion in the 'set' position. This would have shortened the biarticular gastrocnemius, whereas the uniarticular soleus muscle remained in a prestretched position. In both legs, dorsiflexion was observed at the ankle during the early part of the push phase, and thus any activity in the calf muscles was initially eccentric in nature.

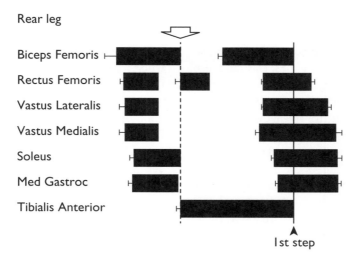

Rear leg

Biceps Femoris

Rectus Femoris

Vastus Lateralis

Vastus Medialis

Soleus

Med Gastroc

Tibialis Anterior

1st step

Fig. 3.5: Duration of electromyographical activity for selected front (A) and rear (B) leg muscles during the block phase and the first two steps of seven trained sprinters (adopted from Guissard and Duchateau, 1990). For each leg, the arrows indicate the instant at which the foot left the block, with the second vertical line indicating the subsequent ground contact with that leg.

Kinematic Aspects

The majority of the kinematic block phase analyses document the joint angles adopted by sprinters when in the 'set' position. These data have been collected from sprinters across a range of abilities, and have thus led to the identification of the positions exhibited by faster sprinters (Mero et al., 1983), as well as the proposition of optimum positioning (Borzov, 1978).

It was suggested by Borzov (1978) that leading sprinters tend to exhibit similar flexion angles in the lower limbs, and thus use different block spacing (that is, inter-block distance, and distance between the front block and the start line) due to differing anthropometrics. Borzov (1978) quoted optimal average values as a front hip angle of 55 degrees, a rear hip angle of 89 degrees, the trunk orientated 14 degrees below the horizontal, a front knee angle of 100 degrees, and

a rear knee angle of 129 degrees, suggesting that when coaching beginners, these angles should be set and the blocks literally placed under the sprinter.

However, Atwater (1982) collected data from a group of eight American national-level sprinters and found trunk angles to range from 9 to 34 degrees below the horizontal, and front knee angles to range between 79 and 112 degrees. This implied that there was a large degree of variation present in 'set' position kinematics, even within a group of international sprinters.

Mero et al. (1983) analysed the starts of twenty-five sprinters (ranged from 10.2 to 11.8sec/100m), and retrospectively divided them into three sub-groups based on their CM velocity at the 2.5m mark. The fastest group (n = 8) were found to adopt smaller angles at both hip joints in the 'set' position. Further tests revealed that these sprinters also had a greater percentage of fast-twitch fibres (sampled from the vastus lateralis), and typically scored more highly on standard strength and power tests such as the squat and counter-movement jumps. This led Mero et al. (1983) to suggest that the between-sprinter differences in 'set' position joint angles may be due to strength differences, with stronger sprinters able to adopt more acute joint angles and to extend the joint over a greater range.

A large amount of kinematic sprint start data was collected from Slovenian national sprinters (males, n = 13, 10.73sec/100m; females, n = 11, 11.97sec/100m) by Čoh et al. (1998). Numerous correlation co-efficients between 'set' position kinematics and performance, quantified as the time taken to reach 5, 10, 20 and 30m (as measured by photocells), were calculated. Results were somewhat inconclusive, with only a handful of moderately strong and statistically significant relationships found.

Whilst the results did suggest that an increased distance between the front block and the start line may be associated with a longer time taken to reach the majority of the measured distances, there were no strong correlations between any of the 'set' position joint angles and any of the performance measures. This again highlights that there is potentially no single optimal position to be adopted in the blocks, and that a large range of 'set' positions exists, independent of the levels of performance achieved.

A potentially more prudent use of the data available to Čoh et al. (1998) would have been to examine how these joint angles changed as the block phase progressed and large forces were generated. In a review of the biomechanics of the sprint start, Harland and Steele (1997) identified seventeen research papers that reported data relating to block positioning and angular kinematics in the 'set' position. In contrast, only three papers were discussed

that related to kinematic aspects of technique during the subsequent block phase.

Two of these were qualitative coaching articles (Hoster and May, 1978; Korchemny, 1992), and one was an experimental investigation altering which leg was placed in the front block (Vagenas and Hoshizaki, 1986). To the author's knowledge, despite the existence of a large body of information regarding 'set' position joint kinematics and the linear kinematics of the CM during block exit, it is still the case that no studies exist which have quantitatively determined how the joint angles change during block exit. There is clearly a greater need for an analysis of technique during the block phase in addition to the abundance of data collected at the very start of this phase. This would increase the understanding of how sprinters achieve the linear impulses and block velocities that are so readily reported.

Kinetic Aspects

Kinetics is the underlying cause of any movement, and several studies have therefore included kinetic analyses in an attempt to further the understanding of the sprint start. Kinematic aspects include the following.

Ground contact and flight time: Mean ground contact times for elite male sprinters have been showed to range from 160 to 194ms for the first ground contact, and 150 to 181ms for the second contact. Mean times for elite sprinters of 60 to 70ms for the first flight, and 44 to 90ms for the second flight have been reported. As is seen, the flight times are considerably less than that spent in the contact phase.

Horizontal velocity: A range of 4.65 to 5.16m/sec for skilled sprinters in the first step and 5.7m/sec for the second post-block step is reported (Harland and Steele, 1997).

Peak force activity: Most studies have combined the forces generated from the front and rear block during the start into singular horizontal, vertical and resultant force components. Maximum total block horizontal, vertical and resultant forces reported for skilled sprinters are ranged from 1186 to 1224N, 766 to 988N and 1426 to 1555N respectively.

Block time: This is defined as the time taken from the beginning of force production, with either foot, to the point where no further force production occurs (that is, the athlete has left the block) and 0.02 to 0.047sec has been reported as the mean value. The front block time demonstrated by skilled sprinters was 0.31 to 0.37sec, with the rear foot pushing for approximately 0.12 to 0.18sec.

Impulse: Impulse incorporates both block force and block time. In fact impulse represents the average amount of force serving to propel the sprinter, and the time over which this force acts. As much horizontal impulse as possible should be attained to enhance start performance.

IMPULSE PRODUCTION

One early kinetic study was undertaken by Baumann (1976), who divided thirty male sprinters into three groups based on 100m performance best times (Group 1: n = 12, mean 10.35 ± 0.12sec/100m; Group 2: n = 8, mean 11.11 ± 0.16sec/100m; Group 3: n = 10, 11.85 ± 0.24sec/100m), and presented a detailed analysis of the recorded force time-histories. The fastest group generated greater total horizontal impulse during the push against the blocks (263 ± 22 Ns) than the other two groups (223 ± 20 Ns and 214 ± 20 Ns, respectively).

As impulse production (relative to mass) determines the change in an object's velocity, and mean masses between groups were similar, the faster group of sprinters thus also achieved higher block velocities (3.6m/sec, compared to 3.1m/sec and 2.9m/sec). The larger impulses of the fastest group were achieved despite spending the same mean amount of time pushing against the blocks as the intermediate group (369ms), and less time than the slowest group (391ms). The increased block velocities of the faster sprinters were therefore due to an increased average horizontal force production, and not to an increase in the duration of the push against the blocks.

Mero et al. (1983) also observed a faster group of sprinters to generate larger horizontal block impulses than their less fast counterparts. Much like the results of Baumann (1976), there were no between-group differences in the duration of force production, thus differences were again due to the mean force generated. This led Mero et al. (1983) to suggest that the level of horizontal force produced is more important than the time taken to produce it. It therefore appears that the ability to generate a large amount of force, without spending overly long doing so, is an important aspect of the block phase.

Some studies have separated the forces generated into those applied against each of the separate blocks, using either two force platforms or strain gauges mounted in each foot plate of the blocks. In a group of seven male sprinters (range from 10.8 to 11.2sec/100m), Guissard and Duchateau (1990) found that larger peak forces were generated at the rear block. However, the rear leg only contributed 24 per cent of the total impulse because the front leg was in contact with the blocks for over twice as long. This concurred with the data of Čoh et al. (2007), where the rear foot was found to contribute only 34 per cent of the total impulse, and thus reinforced the previous suggestions of Payne and Blader (1971) that the front leg is a greater contributor to total impulse.

The importance of the relative contribution of the two legs was highlighted by an experimental investigation in which the dynamic strength of each leg in fifteen trained sprinters was assessed, before a series of sprint start trials was subsequently undertaken (Vagenas and Hoshizaki, 1986). It was found that when the stronger leg was placed in the front block, the group mean block velocity increased to 3.37m/sec from a value of 3.12m/sec when the weaker leg was in the front block. Vagenas and Hoshizaki (1986) attributed these differences to the greater contribution from the front leg to total impulse production.

Although the front leg has a greater contribution to total impulse, it has been suggested that more skilled sprinters actually generate greater peak rear block forces, sometimes also applying less force on the front block than their less skilled counterparts (van Coppenolle et al., 1989; Harland and Steele, 1997; Fortier et al., 2005). From two World Championships finalists, peak rear block forces of 1487 and 1333 N, and peak front block forces of 774 and 1062 N, contributing to total impulses of 301 and 308 Ns, were recorded by van Coppenolle et al. (1989).

These impulse values were associated with block exit velocities of 3.80 and 3.94m/sec respectively. In contrast, these researchers also recorded data from a national level sprinter who exited the blocks with a velocity of 3.34m/sec. Whilst he was able to achieve a similar peak front block force (981 N) to the world class sprinters, his peak force against the rear block was considerably lower (442 N). This led van Coppenolle et al. (1989) to highlight the importance of force generation

with the rear foot during the sprint start, although it must be considered that these kinetic differences may have been due to specific anthropometric or technique factors, rather than ability level.

One further kinetic issue which has previously been highlighted is the angle of force application during block exit. Hafez et al. (1985) identified that although resultant velocity may be higher in one trial, the horizontal component of this velocity was sometimes less than in other analysed trials with lower resultant velocities. Furthermore, whilst horizontal block velocities were found to be greater in those sprinters with quicker PB times, these horizontal block velocities did not appear to be related to the total resultant block force. This supported previous suggestions (Payne and Blader, 1971; Baumann, 1976) that a good start is characterized by the generation of high horizontal impulses, rather than simply high impulses.

This aspect of technique has been associated with the angle between the horizontal and a line joining the CM to the front toe at block exit, which has been found to range between 32 and 42 degrees in well trained sprinters (Mero et al., 1983; Mero, 1988). It has been suggested that provided this angle does not negatively affect the subsequent steps, it should be as low as possible at block exit in order to facilitate horizontal impulse generation (Payne and Blader, 1971).

Block velocities and accelerations: Block velocities for skilled sprinters (10.02 to 10.79sec/100m time) are reported to range from 3.46 to 3.94m/s, and for lesser skilled sprinters from 2.94 to 2.95m/s. Block accelerations for skilled sprinters at the moment of leaving the blocks range from 8.68 to 11.77m/sec^2, and for less skilled sprinters from 6.80 to 7.55m/sec^2 (Harland and Steele, 1977).

IN SUMMARY

Finally, as many variables are introduced pertaining to the block sprint start, the suggestion being that the adaptation of a medium block spacing is preferred with front and rear knee angles in the position approximating 90 and 130 degrees respectively, with the hips moderately high. The sprinter must be capable of developing a high force rate combined with a high maximum force, especially in the horizontal direction.

The ability to create high force underlies other important indicators of starting performance, such as minimum block clearance time, maximum block-leaving velocity and maximum block-leaving acceleration. Once the sprinter has projected him/herself from the block at a low angle (40 to 45 degrees) relative to the ground, the following two post-block steps should occur with the total body centre of mass ahead of the contacting foot at foot strike in order to minimize horizontal braking forces, therefore increasing sprinter horizontal velocity.

CHAPTER 4

BIOMECHANICS OF SPRINTING

by Professor Morteza Shahbazi Moghaddam

We discussed the meaning of biomechanics and sprinting in the last chapter. We also looked at the technique of the sprint start. We shall now move on to the acceleration phase and to cruising at top speed.

THE RUNNING CYCLE

In running there are four main phases:

Phase I: Initial contact (braking) – this is the first contact that the foot makes with the ground: this may be the heel, the whole of the foot at once, or the front of the foot (forefoot).

Phase II: Mid-stance – at this point the whole body is balancing on one leg. The entire foot is usually in contact with the ground, and the other leg is swinging through.

Phase III: Propulsion – the supporting leg leaves the ground before the opposite leg comes into contact with the floor.

Phase IV: Swing – the non-supporting leg swings past the stationary leg ready for the next step.

All these phases differ depending on the running style and speed. Generally there are two different fast running styles, depending on the speed of the runner, which are characterized in the table (below).

SPRINTING GAIT CYCLE

The gait cycle starts when one of the feet makes contact with the ground, and ends when that same foot makes contact with the ground again. It can be divided up into two 'phases': the stance phase, during which the foot is in contact with the ground, and the swing phase, during which the foot is not in contact with the ground.

The stance phase is typically considered to be the more important of the two, as it is when the foot and leg bear the bodyweight. The swing phase is passive because it is not consciously controlled. Trying to actively help the leg move through the swing phase – by consciously trying to lift the front knee higher, or trying to lift the heel higher towards the backside – is an example of where sprinters waste energy.

THE RUNNING CYCLE AND STYLE

Style of running	Initial Contact	Mid-stance	Propulsion	Swing
Sprinting	This is usually made with the front of the foot. The heel may touch the ground later (or not), depending on the individual running style	This phase is very rapid and the foot is usually in the same position as in initial contact	The hips extend back ready to propel the runner forwards for take-off. The arms swing at full power to help	The non-supporting leg swings high with the knee at almost a 90-degree angle
Fast running	Most fast runners will make initial contact with the middle of their foot or heel	Only a very short amount of time will be spent in mid-stance as the runner pushes through with his foot	Push-off is through the big toe, with the runner's hips extended back and his knee slightly bent	The knee of the runner's non-supporting leg will be lifted, although not as high as with a sprint

The Stance Phase

This phase can be divided into four stages: initial contact, braking (absorption), mid-stance and propulsion.

Initial contact: At the moment of the stride and when both feet are off the floor (sometimes referred to as the float phase), if the right leg is out in front of the sprinter and about to touch the ground, this moment (whether the sprinter lands on the heel, midfoot, or forefoot) is called the initial contact and marks the beginning of the stance phase. The left foot behind the sprinter is off the floor and in the swing phase. See Fig. 4.1 (a).

Braking (absorption): As soon as the left foot makes contact with the ground in front of the sprinter, the sprinter's body is, in effect, performing a controlled landing, managed through deceleration and braking. The left knee and ankle flex and the left foot rolls in (prorates) to absorb the impact forces. During this process of absorption, the tendons and connective tissue within the muscles store elastic energy for use later in the propulsion phase. See Fig. 4.1 (c) and (d).

Mid-stance: The braking phase above continues until the left leg is directly under the hips taking the maximum load (with a maximum risk of injury) as the bodyweight passes over it. The left ankle and knee are at the angle of maximum flexion. This moment is called midstance or the single support phase. See Fig. 4.1 (c).

Propulsion: Now that the left leg has made a controlled landing and absorbed as much energy as it is going to get, it starts to propel the sprinter forwards. This is achieved by the left hip, knee and ankle all extending (straightening) to push the body up and forwards, using the elastic energy stored during the braking phase above. The more elastic energy available at this stage, the less the body has to use the muscles.

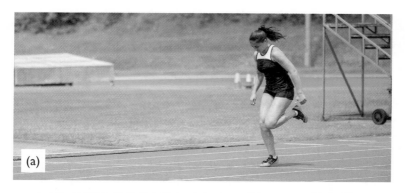

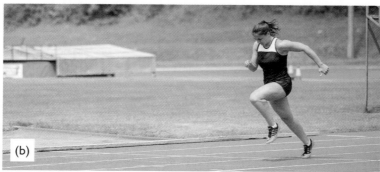

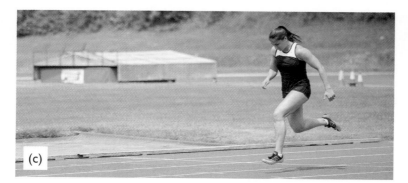

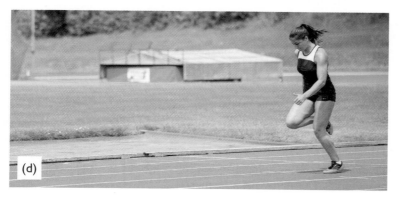

Fig. 4.1 (a–d): Sprinter showing the propulsion, mid-stance, swing and braking phases. (Photos: Darren Charles Holloway)

The propulsion phase ends when the toe of the left foot (now behind the sprinter) leaves the ground, commonly referred to as the 'toe off'. At this point, both feet are off the ground so that the sprinter is once again in the float phase. See Fig. 4.1 (d).

The Swing Phase

At the moment of 'toe off', the left leg has travelled as far back as it is going to, and the heel starts to lift towards the backside. As was mentioned earlier, this is a passive movement (as opposed to a conscious effort), with the height that the heel reaches depending on the degree of hip extension achieved and the speed at which the sprinter is running.

If you compare this stretch reflex mechanism to stretching back a sling shot and then letting it go, the extension of the hip (as the back leg moves behind the sprinter prior to 'toe off') is equivalent to pulling back on the sling shot. Letting go results in the leg firing forwards rapidly, leading with the knee. Any conscious attempt to move the leg through the swing phase, which can also be referred to as the 'recovery phase', results in wasted energy and a less powerful firing of the sling shot. Once the knee has passed under the hip, the lower leg unfolds in preparation, once again for initial contact, marking the end of the swing phase – see Fig. 4.1 (a) to (c).

The Return Phase

The return phase begins when the foot strikes the ground in front of the sprinter, and ends when the knee and thigh of the same foot are perpendicular to the ground directly beneath him/her (see Fig. 4.2). This is the shortest of all the phases and is often overlooked. However, it has a huge impact on sprinting speed, where $1/100$ of a second can mean the difference between winning and losing.

The Push Phase

Many people associate the push phase (see Fig. 4.3) with the first few steps at the start of the race, where the body is lowest to the ground, as it comes out of the starting blocks, and where this phase is dominant. However, the push phase, just like the other

**Fig. 4.2 (a–c):
The return phase.
(Photos: Darren
Charles Holloway)**

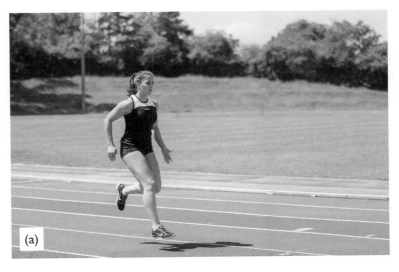

(a)

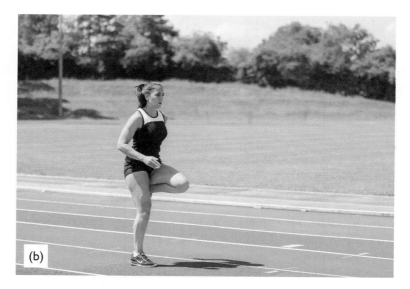

(b)

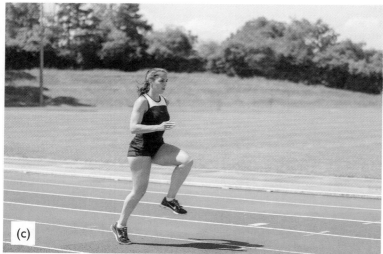

(c)

Fig. 4.2 (a–c)
(*continued*)

two phases, occurs throughout the entire running process, even while the body is upright. Since the body is upright for most of the time and certainly for the distance that the sprinter spends running, the push phase will be addressed while the body is in its upright position. The push phase begins when the thigh of the foot touching the ground is perpendicular to the ground, and it ends when the toes of this foot have just left the ground behind the sprinter.

Upper Body and Arm Mechanics

Driving the elbows down as well as back can help to avoid elevation of the shoulders. The interaction between the upper and lower body plays a vital role in running, the upper body and arm action providing balance and promoting efficient movement. This balance is achieved by the arms and upper body effectively working in direct opposition to the legs. Bringing the left arm forwards opposes

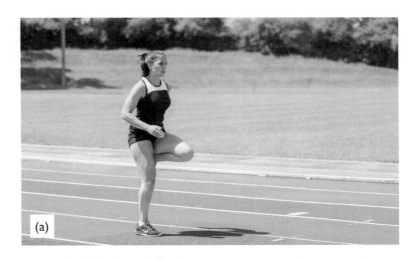

(a)

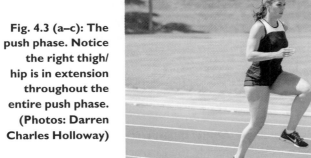

Fig. 4.3 (a–c): The push phase. Notice the right thigh/hip is in extension throughout the entire push phase. (Photos: Darren Charles Holloway)

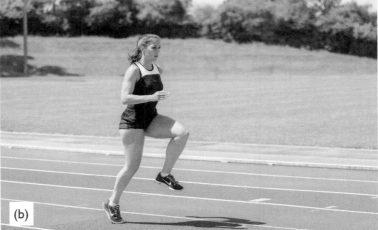

(b)

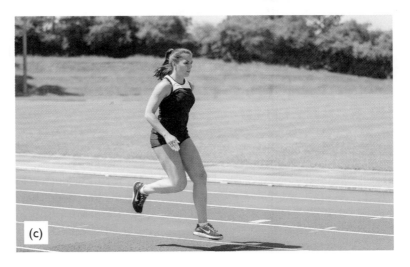

(c)

the forward drive of the right leg, and vice versa. During the braking (absorption) stage described above (initial contact to mid-stance), the arms and upper body produce a propulsive force.

During the propulsion stage (mid-stance to toe off), the arms and upper body produce a braking force.

By working as opposites, forward momentum is maintained. The arms and upper body also counterbalance rotation in the mid-section. For example, as the right knee is fired through in front of the body (the right swing phase), an anticlockwise momentum is created. To counterbalance this, the left arm and shoulder move forwards to create a clockwise momentum to reduce rotational forces.

To help the above occur as efficiently as possible, the arm swing should be initiated at and through the shoulders, which in itself causes tightness and limits range of motion. Just as bringing the knee through in the swing phase needs to be a passive movement, so does the forward movement of the arm. Driving the arms up and forwards wastes energy and reduces the efficiency of the stretch reflex mechanism in the shoulders. The hands crossing the mid-line of the body is a sign that the sprinter may be driving the arms forwards instead of backwards, or that he/she has tightness in the chest.

MUSCLES INVOLVED IN SPRINTING

There are several groups of muscles in the lower and upper limbs involved in different phases of sprinting.

Muscles Involved in the Push Phase

The muscles involved in the push phase (from mid-stance to toe off) are the following:

Knee extensors (quadriceps): These include rectus femoris, vastus medialis, vastus lateralis and vastus intermedius. These muscles provide for leg extension at the knee. (The rectus femoris also provides for thigh/hip flexion, however thigh flexion is not part of the push phase, but rather the swing phase.)

Thigh/hip extensor muscles: These include the gluteus maximus muscle and the hamstrings. Most people associate the hamstrings strictly with flexing the leg behind the thigh, however they are also very powerful thigh/hip extensors. The hamstrings involved in thigh/hip extension are semimembranosus, semitendinosus, and the long head of the biceps femoris. Note that the short head of the biceps femoris does not act to extend the hip/thigh.

Ankle flexors (the calf muscles): These include the gastrocnemius, soleus and plantaris muscles. These provide plantar flexion of the foot.

Muscles Involved in the Swing Phase

The three muscle groups involved in the swing phase are as follows:

THIGH FLEXORS

Also known as hip flexors, these muscles include the psoas, iliacus, sartorius, vastus rectus, adductor longis, adductor brevis and the pectineus. These muscles flex the thigh on the pelvis, as shown in Fig. 4.5.

Collectively as a group, the thigh flexors are among the strongest muscle groups in

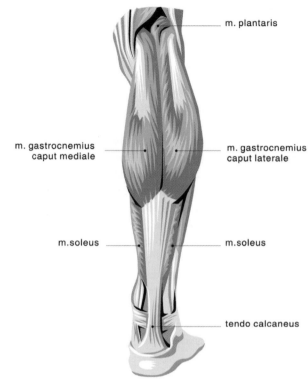

Fig. 4.4: The calf muscles. (Shutterstock)

m. plantaris

m. gastrocnemius caput mediale

m. gastrocnemius caput laterale

m.soleus

m.soleus

tendo calcaneus

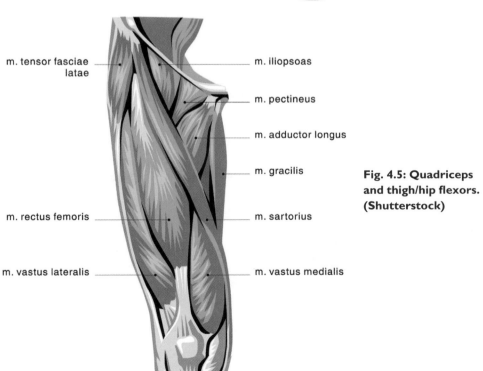

m. tensor fasciae latae

m. iliopsoas

m. pectineus

m. adductor longus

m. gracilis

m. rectus femoris

m. sartorius

m. vastus lateralis

m. vastus medialis

Fig. 4.5: Quadriceps and thigh/hip flexors. (Shutterstock)

the body. They are responsible for performing such functions as controlling posture, sitting, standing, walking, running and jumping.

QUADRICEPS

These include the vastus rectus, vastus medialis, vastus lateralis and the vastus intermedius (see Fig. 4.5).

The quadriceps' function is to extend the leg at the knee. When the lower leg is flexed behind, the thigh will then be extended at the thigh preparing for the ground touchdown. While leg extension is important during this phase, the relative strength of the quadriceps is not fully appreciated here, since leg extension during this motion takes place with the leg off the ground, or in a non-weight-bearing position. The quadriceps, therefore, contribute more during the push phase when the foot is on the ground, than they do during the swing phase when the foot is in the air.

HAMSTRINGS

These include the semimembranosus, semitendinosus and biceps femoris (long and short heads) (see Fig. 4.6).

The hamstrings play a very limited role in the swing phase. Their only function during this phase is leg flexion (or knee flexion). However, as can be seen, leg flexion (leg flexing behind the thigh) has very little to do with running. The real value of hamstrings, with respect to running, is their ability to provide for powerful thigh/hip extension, which makes up a big part of the push phase and the return phase.

Muscles Involved in the Return Phase

This is the return phase of running in its most basic form. The following muscles are involved in the return phase:

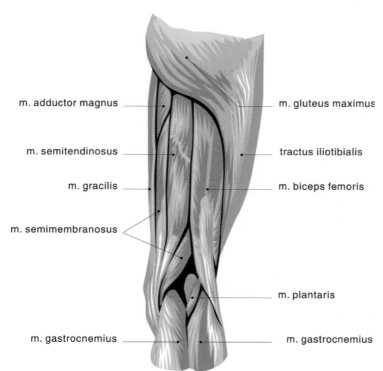

m. adductor magnus

m. semitendinosus

m. gracilis

m. semimembranosus

m. gastrocnemius

m. gluteus maximus

tractus iliotibialis

m. biceps femoris

m. plantaris

m. gastrocnemius

Fig. 4.6: Hamstrings and thigh/hip extensor. (Shutterstock)

THE THIGH EXTENSOR MUSCLES

These include the gluteus maximus, semi-membranosus, semitendinosus and the biceps femoris (long head); the semimembranosus, semitendinosus and biceps femoris (long head) are also known as the hamstring muscles (see Fig. 4.6).

In fact the hamstring muscles have *two* functions: leg flexion, as seen during the swing phase, and thigh extension, as seen in this return phase as well as the push phase. And between the two, the ability of the hamstrings to extend the thighs plays a much more significant role in athletics than does their ability to flex the legs. Thigh extension, along with thigh flexion (swing phase), are sprinter power-generating motions, and improving these will enable the athlete to reap huge rewards in performance. Leg flexion (hamstrings), on the other hand, is a motion that typically follows after the power moves, similar to a recoil, or a change in momentum, after the muscular energy is spent. This was seen in the swing phase where the leg was flexed behind the thigh.

It may be noticed from Fig. 4.2 that the position (angle) of the right leg relative to the right thigh doesn't change all that much in the rest of the figures. In other words, the leg does not really flex all that much behind the thigh while the foot is on the ground throughout this motion. The real change is seen in the position of the right thigh. In fact, the right thigh is really extending and showing a function of the gluteus maximus and hamstrings.

By going through extension, the thigh (since it is in front of the sprinter) helps to pull the sprinter body forwards. That is why the return phase is sometimes referred to as the pull phase, because of the pulling effect the hamstrings have on the thigh. It is also where the phrase 'pulled a hamstring' comes from, since it is during this motion or during the transition from the swing phase to the return phase that the hamstrings are often injured. Though its importance in speed is limited, keeping sprinter hamstring muscles strong and flexible will help prevent injury to this muscle.

MOVEMENT IN THE HIP AND KNEE JOINTS

As sprint running is extremely technical, it involves therefore the use and coordination of the entire body. Olympic sprinters finely tune the biomechanics of their sprint running form for years to reduce their times by fractions of a second. We will see how muscles in these joints contract either eccentrically or concentrically in four basic phases of sprint running: in eccentric motion, tension increases on the muscle as it lengthens. In concentric motion, tension increases on the muscle as it shortens. For example, biceps muscle is undergoing eccentric muscle flexion – bending motion – during the downward phase of a biceps curl, and concentric muscle flexion during the upward phase.

The Initial Phase

The last milliseconds before the foot makes contact with the ground is when the initial phase occurs. This phase involves two major motions: concentric hip extension and eccentric knee flexion. The concentric hip extension movement is responsible for rotating the thigh backwards. This balances the body over the feet, allowing the sprinter to take his/her next step. The eccentric knee flexion accelerates the entire leg backwards. This motion limits the knee extension and helps to minimize braking when the sprinter foot reaches the ground.

The Mid-Stance Phase

This phase takes only milliseconds and is the most basic of the phases. One major motion occurs during this phase, and that is concentric hip flexion. During concentric hip flexion, the sprinter is accelerating his/her thigh forward. The concentric hip flexion phase is where the sprinter prepares for the next propulsive step to occur.

The Swing Phase

During the swing phase, the hips and knees do the majority of the work. They are preparing for the next step in the stride. Two movements occur during this phase: eccentric hip flexion and eccentric knee extension. During eccentric hip flexion the sprinter is decelerating the backward rotation of the thigh. The eccentric knee extension motion involves the quadriceps muscles, which act to slow the backward rotation of the leg and foot.

The Push Phase

This phase is responsible for forward propulsion, and several movements occur in it. The first is eccentric hip flexion, which is responsible for slowing the backward thigh rotation. The next is concentric knee extension, a straightening motion that propels the centre of mass forwards. The last motion to occur is concentric plantar flexion, which gives the sprinter forward propulsion.

MUSCLES INVOLVED IN THE UPPER BODY

The upper body muscles such as the abdominis, brachi, brachialis and brachiora-

dialis are also involved in sprinting in order to coordinate the movement of the sprinter in his performance (see Figs 4.8 and 4.9).

Posture and Stability

Posture is a key part of sprinting form: sprinters burst out of the starting blocks while leaning forward, then gradually assume an upright position. For longer sprints, in particular, it is vital to maintain an erect posture for most of the race. The core muscles most responsible for establishing and holding the correct posture include the rectus abdominus at the front of the abdomen, the obliques and transverse abdominus at the sides, and the erector spinae in the lower back (see Fig. 4.10).

Elbow Flexion

Sprinters bend their elbows as they leave the blocks at the start of a sprint race, and they maintain that elbow bend as they pump their arms for the remainder of the sprint. The upper arm muscles – primarily the biceps brachii, brachialis and brachioradialis – are responsible for elbow flexion.

KINEMATICS

The sprinter's goal is to develop the highest possible horizontal velocity. For elite sprinters this velocity is developed over the course of the forty-three to forty-six strides (men) and forty-seven to fifty-two strides (women) that make up the 100m race. The sprinter's horizontal propulsion is only produced during the support phase. The support leg applies force against the ground in a backward downward direction (the action), and the ground reaction results in horizontal propulsion in a forward upward direction.

There is only a little time available for the sprinter to apply force during the support phase. At the point of maximum velocity, the foot is only on the ground for 0.08–0.09sec during the support phase, so the sprinter must be able to apply force effectively during this short time period to maintain horizontal velocity. This alone highlights the necessity of sprinters having the ability to apply a large amount of force in a very short time period.

Mathematically, velocity is the product of stride length and stride frequency:

velocity = stride length × stride frequency

Fig. 4.7 (a–c): Concentric hip extension, eccentric knee flexion, eccentric hip flexion and eccentric knee extension, concentric knee extension and concentric plantar flexion are demonstrated by the sprinter. Notice how the knee is responsible for absorbing the strike. (Photos: Darren Charles Holloway)

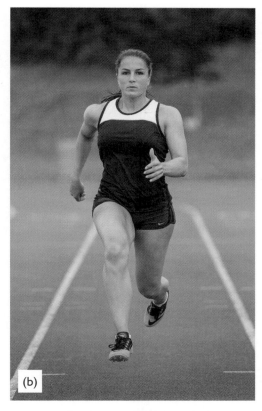
(b)

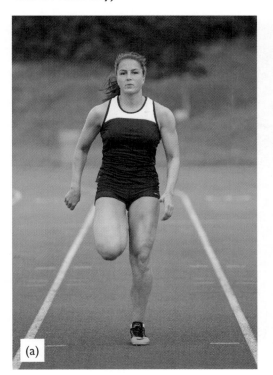
(a)

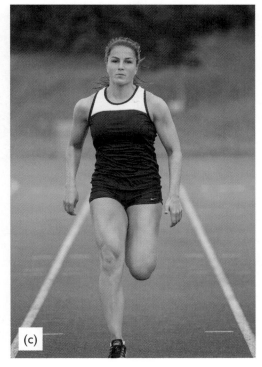
(c)

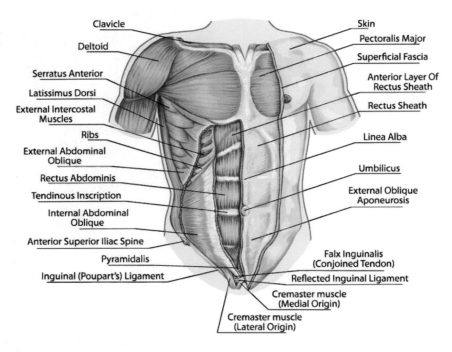

Fig. 4.8: Rectus and transverse abdominus muscles. (Shutterstock)

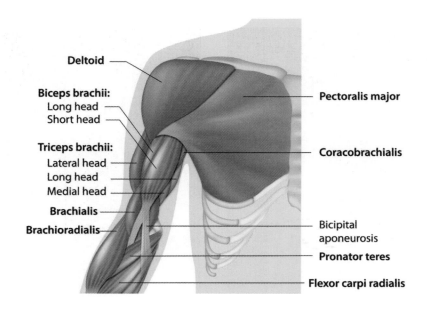

Fig. 4.9: Brachialis and brachioradialis muscles. (Shutterstock)

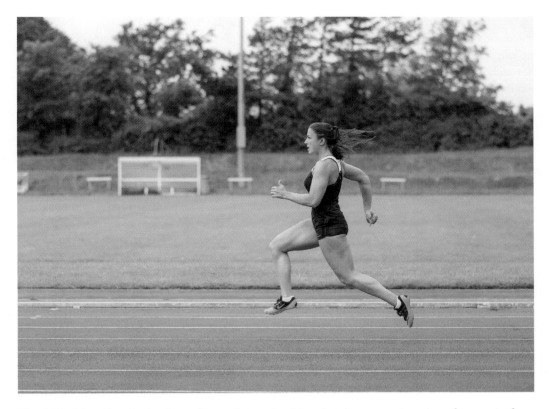

Fig. 4.10: After the start release the sprinter should maintain an erect posture for most of the race. (Photo: Darren Charles Holloway)

These two factors interact in the 100m, and after they have reached a certain point following a phase in which they mutually increase (within the first 50m), an increase in either parameter will result in a corresponding decrease in the other. This part in the race depends on many factors, such as body type, power production, training status and fatigue level, and is individual to each athlete. There is therefore an optimal stride length and frequency for each athlete. In fact, five biomechanical factors in sprinting can be considered:

■ The reaction phase at the start
■ The acceleration phase (increase in velocity)
■ The maximum velocity phase (constant velocity)
■ The deceleration phase (decreasing velocity)
■ The finish

As was mentioned in the previous chapter, during the reaction phase the sprinter uses the resistance of the start blocks to accelerate initially from a complete rest position. An explosive force production of the legs in a very short time is vital for a successful start. After the start signal the sprinter must develop horizontal forces reaching up to 1.5 times his bodyweight in less than 0.4sec. The reaction time (the time between the start signal to the first movement of the sprinter) is of relatively small importance to the overall result (relative to the other phases of the race). Average reaction time values for elite sprinters range from 0.12–0.18sec, which constitutes only 1–2 per cent of the total 100m (the percentage is even smaller for slower sprinters).

After leaving the start blocks the sprinter increases his running speed in the acceleration phase by continually increasing stride length and stride frequency. This segment begins with full block clearance, and concludes when there is no further positive change in velocity. Depending on the sprinter's level of ability, this segment occurs from approximately 2m to 25–50m (Shahbazi et al. 2002 (a)). The greater the velocity developed by the sprinter, the longer the acceleration phase, although maximum speed is usually realized within 4–5sec after the start, regardless of the maximum speed generated (Shahbazi et al. 2002 (b)).

During this phase men achieve stride frequencies of up to 4.6 strides per second, and women 4.8 strides per second. The length of the acceleration phase increases at higher performance levels, and this is the most important phase for the race performance. Top sprinters reach their maximum speed after about 45–60m (men) and 40–50m (women).

In the phase of maximum speed (at 50–80m) the sprinters cover a distance of 20–30m at their highest velocity. This segment begins when there is no further positive change in velocity, and concludes when a negative change in velocity begins (see Fig. 4.16. This is where the maximum speeds of 12m/s (men) and 11m/s (women) are achieved. Stride length and stride frequency vary among sprinters, and each will have an optimal ratio for maximum velocity. This is also the phase where the ground contact times are the shortest.

The final 10–20m constitutes the deceleration phase. This phase begins when a negative change in velocity is seen, and ends two to four strides before the finish line. The length of this segment is dependent on the length of the acceleration and maximum velocity segment. Fatigue leads to a decreased stride frequency, for which the sprinter attempts to compensate by increasing the stride length.

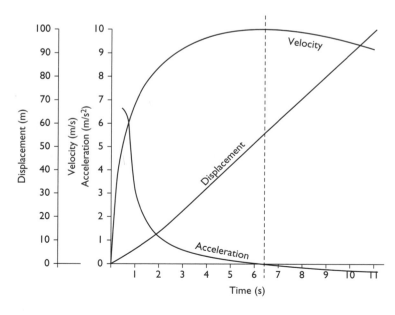

Fig. 4.11: Adapted from *An Introduction to the Mechanics of Human Movements* by James Watkins, 1983. Variations of displacement, velocity and acceleration for a typical sprinter are depicted.

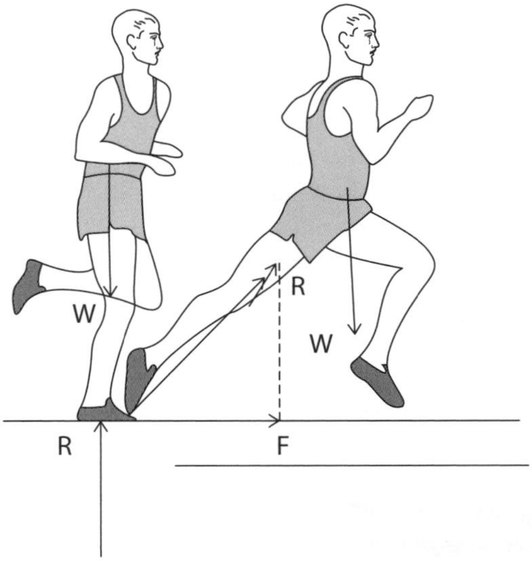

Fig. 4.12: At the pushing phase the sprinter produces an external force with two components. The horizontal component propels the sprinter in a forward direction.

The finish (the final two to four strides) is the decisive stage of the race, especially between sprinters with minimal differences in ability. Competition rules state that the clock stops when the trunk of the body passes the finish line, so a strong forward lean is an advantage to the sprinter. This can be achieved by flexing the hips while simultaneously swinging back the arms.

FATIGUE

Fatigue is a prominent factor in sprinting. It is already widely known that it hinders maximal power output in muscles, but it also affects the acceleration of runners in the ways listed below.

Submaximal Muscle Coordination

A study on muscle coordination in which subjects performed repeated 6sec cycling sprints, or intermittent sprints of short duration (ISSD), showed a correlation between a decrease in maximal power output and changes in motor coordination. In this case, motor coordination refers to the ability to coordinate muscle movements in order to optimize a physical action, so submaximal coordination indicates that the muscles are no longer activating 'in sync' with one another.

The results of the study showed a delay in coordination between the vastus lateralis (VL) and the biceps femoris (BF) muscles. Since there was a decrease in power during ISSD occurring in tandem with changes in VL-BF coordination, it is indicated that changes in inter-muscle coordination is one of the contributing factors for the reduced power output resulting from fatigue. This was done using bicycle sprinting, but the principles carry over to sprinting from a runner's perspective.

Hindrance of Effective Force Application Techniques

Morin *et al.* (2005) explored the effects of fatigue on force production and force application techniques in a study where sprinters performed four sets of five 6sec sprints using the same treadmill set-up as previously mentioned. Data was collected on their ability to produce ground reaction forces as well as their ability to coordinate the ratio of ground forces (horizontal to vertical) to allow for greater horizontal acceleration.

The immediate results showed a significant decrease in performance with each sprint, and a sharper decrease in the rate of performance depreciation with each subsequent data set. In conclusion, it was obvious that both the total force production capability and the technical ability to apply ground forces were greatly affected.

KINETICS

The kinetics of running describes the motion of a runner using the effects of forces acting on or out of the body. The majority of contributing factors to internal forces comes from leg muscle activation and arm swing.

Leg Muscle Activation

The muscles responsible for accelerating the runner forwards are required to contract with increasing speed to accommodate the increasing velocity of the body. During the acceleration phase of sprinting, the contractile component of muscles is the main component responsible for the power output. Once a steady state velocity has been reached and the sprinter is upright, a sizable fraction of the power comes from the mechanical energy stored in the 'series elastic elements' during stretching of the contractile muscles that is released immediately after the positive work phase. As the velocity of the runner increases, inertia and air-resistance effects become the limiting factors on the sprinter's top speed.

It was previously believed that there was an intramuscular viscous force that increased proportionally to the velocity of muscle contraction that opposed the contractile force; however, this theory has since been disproved.

Arm Swing

Arm swing occurs from the shoulders, so that the shoulders do not turn or sway. It is a simple, pendulum-like forward and backward motion without shoulder sway and without crossing the arms in front of the body. On the forward upswing the arm angle should decrease slightly, with the hands in a relaxed fist. On the backswing they should swing back to just above and behind the hip joint for most running speeds. As the running speed increases, the arm will swing back more, eventually culminating in going back and upwards in sprinting.

Contrary to the findings of Mann et al. (1981), arm swing plays a vital role in both stabilizing the torso and vertical propulsion. Regarding torso stabilization, arm swing serves to counterbalance the rotational momentum created by leg swing, as suggested by Hinrichs et al. (1987). In short, the athlete would have a hard time controlling the rotation of their trunk without arm swing. Jones et al. (2009) and Mann et al. (2008), and Čoh et al. (2006) documented the arms' balancing function in relation to the motion of the legs while sprinting with the elbow angle maintained at close to 90 degrees of flexion. The arms should work as a balancing factor by providing lift and promoting a more horizontal velocity for the runner.

The same study also suggested that, as opposed to popular belief, the horizontal force production capabilities of the arms are limited due to the backward swing that follows the forward swing, so the two components cancel each other out. This is not to suggest, however, that arm swing does not

Fig. 4.13: The horizontal component is in a forward direction in start, but is in the opposite direction at finish.

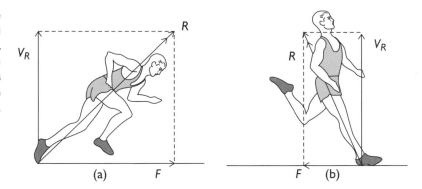

(a)   (b)

contribute to propulsion at all during sprinting; in fact, it can contribute up to 10 per cent of the total vertical propulsive forces that a sprinter can apply to the ground. The reason for this is that, unlike the forward-backward motion, both arms are synchronized in their upward-downward movement. As a result, there is no cancellation of forces.

Forces Generated During Sprinting

Referring to Fig. 4.13, at the standing phase, the only forces acting on the sprinter are bodyweight, W, and the ground reaction force, R, which is equal and opposite to W such that the resultant force on him is zero. In the pushing phase, the sprinter creates an external force that acts on his/her body in the direction of run.

The ground reaction force always has a vertical component which counteracts bodyweight. The magnitude and direction of the ground reaction and, therefore, of V_R and F, will depend upon the type of activity. In the sprint start, for example, the athlete wants to generate maximum velocity forwards, and consequently, the horizontal component (which is also called frictional force) of the ground reaction will be relatively large and in the direction of run – see Fig. 4.14 (a). However, when the sprinter slows down at the end of the race,

the frictional force will act in the opposite direction since it is then the decelerating force – see Fig. 4.14 (b).

The force that drives the sprinter forwards is the propulsive force F, and running speed is directly related to the magnitude of this force. An Olympic sprinter can push off the ground with a total peak force of more than 1,000lb (with a time-averaged F equal to about 200lb, which is less than the peak F). In contrast, the average runner can apply 500–600lb of total peak force. According to Weyand et al. (2000), during a sprint the average sprinter's foot is on the ground for about 0.12sec, while an Olympic sprinter's foot is on the ground for just 0.08sec.

Path Travelled by the Runner's Centre of Mass

As the sprinter runs along, his centre of mass follows a parabolic arc, as shown in Fig. 4.19. This parabolic path is due to the force of gravity acting on the sprinter between his foot strikes with the ground. These foot strikes propel him through the air in a shallow arc, up until the time he lands with his other foot, at which point he pushes off the ground with that foot, which then sends him once more through the air with his centre of mass following a parabolic arc. The force with which the runner pushes off the ground serves as an initial launch force, which causes his centre of mass to follow a parabolic arc, as is explained by Newton's second law and the equations of projectile motion. The greater the force F, the greater the horizontal running velocity, and the longer the arc length, hence the faster the sprinter will run.

centre of mass moves
in parabolic arcs

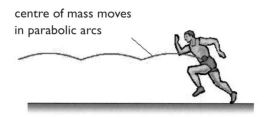

Fig. 4.14: The parabolic movement of the sprinter's centre of mass.

CHAPTER 5

BIOMECHANICS OF SUNDRY SPRINT SKILLS

by Professor Morteza Shahbazi Moghaddam

We discussed the meaning of biomechanics and sprinting, as well as the technique of the sprint start, in Chapter 3. We covered the skills involved in sprinting, that is accelerating to full speed and cruising at top speed in a straight line, in Chapter 4. We will now consider a few sundry skills that sprinters require in order to be good team members. These skills include the dip finish that may assist a sprinter to win a race, curve running around bends, running slightly further than we can manage flat out anaerobically, and running relays.

THE DIP FINISH

Running at the highest level is incredibly technical, but even the top athletes make basic errors of judgement that cost them medals. Some athletes fail to relax so they tense up in the heat of battle, others make a sluggish start or, worse still, bolt from the blocks too early so they are disqualified from the race. But one of the most agonizing sights in the sport remains seeing an athlete dominate a race, put him or herself in a perfect position to clinch glory, only to throw it all away by failing to dip at the line and have victory snatched from them by someone who did.

While there is some difficulty in timing the lunge towards the line perfectly, failing

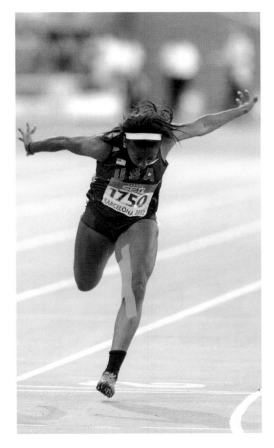

Fig. 5.1: Dipping is the sprinter's last attempt to secure a medal. (Photo: Shutterstock)

to do so altogether can be fairly regarded as negligent when it comes to performing at the highest level. There are numerous examples of athletes at major championships losing out on gold, silver or bronze by simply running through the line and not dipping.

As Britain's victorious Christine Ohuruogu proved in the women's 400m final at the 2013 World Championships, a strong finish with a well timed dip can be the crucial difference between glory and the intense frustration of a near-but-not-quite second place. Ohuruogu beat defending champion Amantle Montsho in a photo finish. Both finished in 49.41 seconds, but the Brit's late dip saw her triumph by four thousandths of a second.

The 2007 world champion also broke Kathy Cook's long-standing British record by two hundredths of a second, but none of it would have been achieved had she not dipped desperately at the line. A distraught Montsho was left utterly stunned after Ohuruogu was announced as the winner, and as former GB athlete Colin Jackson told the BBC after the race, 'She will never forgive herself for not winning that race'. It was almost tragic, but entirely her fault. Montsho had victory well within her grasp until she failed to dip at the line, which saw her finish in 49.408 with Ohuruogu's last-gasp lunge seeing her home in 49.404.

Coming off the final turn in the men's 400m hurdles final, Gordon trailed American Michael Tinsley, but recalling advice from his mother and coach, he claimed a dramatic victory by ensuring that he was the athlete who successfully dipped at the line (see Fig. 5.2).

CURVE RUNNING

Sprinting round a turn – see Fig. 5.3 – (such as for the 200m and 400m races) is known to result in a longer race time than if the race were run on a straight track. This is due to the centrifugal force ($F_c = mv^2/R$) experienced by the sprinter as he goes round the turn, which has the effect of diminishing the force

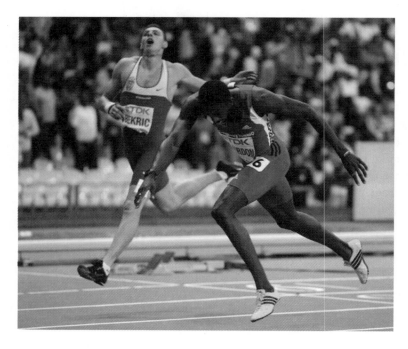

Fig. 5.2: My head actually left my body and went over the line, and my body went behind it and won gold as a result.

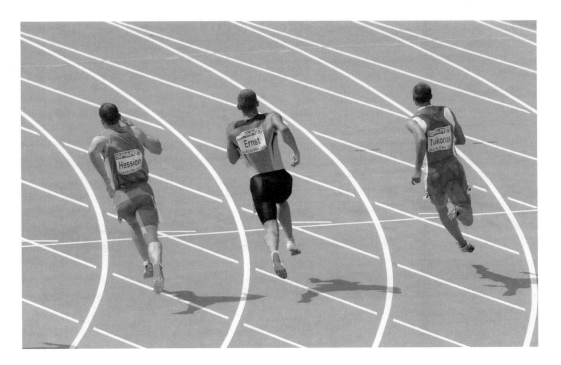

Fig. 5.3: Centrifugal force (in an outward direction relative to the centre of the turn) makes sprinters apply the same amount of force (in an inward direction) in order to run in their track. (Photo: Shutterstock)

available to him for propelling himself round the track. As expected, this effect is more pronounced the smaller the turn radius is, and as a result we have the common complaint by runners that the inside lane is 'too tight'. Fig. 5.4 shows the contact forces acting between the runner's foot and the curved track. The turn radius is R.

Fig. 5.4: F_c is an extra force provided, in addition to push-off force F_t, by the sprinter to maintain his/her curved running path round the track. The resultant force makes him bend outwards while turning. Running round a turn forces the runner to produce a centrifugal force F_c in order to maintain his/her curved running path round the track. This centrifugal force is in addition to the force necessary to propel him tangentially along the track, which is F_t. The total force F (exerted by the runner on the track) has components F_t and F_c.

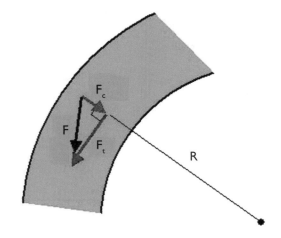

Alexandrov and Lucht (1981) determine that a runner in lane 1 (the innermost lane) would run the 200m in 19.72sec, whereas in lane 8 (the outermost lane) he would run it in 19.60sec. This is a big time difference, and translates into a distance of about one metre at the finish line. Since many races are won or lost by mere centimetres, this is a very significant difference. However, it should be pointed out that sprinters do not consider lane 8 to be the most advantageous one either, since, due to the staggered starts, they would run half the race ahead of the other runners, which puts them at a psychological disadvantage because they are not able to see what the others are doing.

At major events it is usual for the participants to be seeded so that those who run the faster times in the heats are awarded the inner lanes in the next round, and those who run the slower times are awarded the outer lanes.

RUNNING 400 METRES

According to an analysis given by Keller (1973) and based on the physiology of record holders from 1973, the runner should accelerate as fast as possible for 1.78sec. This will enable him to reach a speed near his maximum. He should then maintain this speed for as long as he can. This speed will be such that 0.86sec before the end of the race his energy is entirely used up, and after this point is reached his running speed will begin to drop. Clearly this would be difficult to reproduce exactly in an actual race, but it does give some non-intuitive insight into how 400m sprinters might maximize their performance. Fig. 5.5 illustrates this for a typical 400m men's race.

Where t_1 and t_2 are intermediate times representing the start and end of the cruising (constant speed) stage, T is the time at which the race ends. Now, $t_1 = 1.78$sec, and $t_2 = T-0.86$sec. This is based on the physiology of record holders from 1973. The numbers 1, 2, 3 represent the three stages of the race: the acceleration stage (1), the cruising stage (2), and the deceleration stage (3).

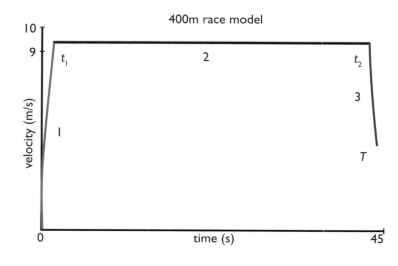

400m race model

Fig. 5.5: In contrast to 100m sprinting, in a 400m course the constant speed takes place over a very long time, while acceleration and deceleration period times are very short.

THE SPRINT RELAY

The 4 × 100m relay, or sprint relay, is an athletics track event run in lanes over one lap of the track with four runners completing 100m each. The aim of the 100m sprint relay is, with the assistance of four athletes, to carry a baton (30cm long, 13cm in circumference and no less than 50g in weight) around 400m as quickly as possible.

The four runners begin in the same stagger as for the individual 400m race. The relay baton is carried by each runner and must be passed within a 20m changeover box (usually marked by yellow lines), which extends 10m on either side of each 100m mark of the race. Another line is marked 10m further back, marking the earliest point at which the outgoing runner may begin (giving up to 10m of acceleration before entering the passing zone).

Transferring the baton in this race is typically blind. The outgoing runner reaches a straight arm backwards when they enter the changeover box, or when the incoming runner makes a verbal signal (see Fig. 5.6). The outgoing runner does not look backwards, and it is the responsibility of the incoming runner to thrust the baton into the outstretched hand, and not let go until the outgoing runner takes hold of it.

Runners on the first and third legs typically run on the inside of the lane with the baton in their right hand, while runners on the second and fourth legs take the baton in their left. Polished handovers can compensate for a lack of basic speed to some extent, and disqualification for dropping the baton or failing to transfer it within the box is common, even at the highest level.

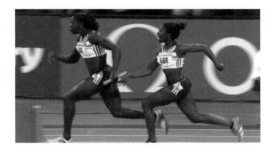

Fig. 5.6: The outgoing runner receiving the baton securely in the changeover box, after the incoming runner also made a verbal signal.

Running Line and Baton Exchange

The rules of relay competition require the baton to be exchanged within a 20m changeover zone so that the outgoing runner can achieve maximum acceleration at baton exchange. The athlete can commence his/her run 10m before the changeover zone. The baton exchange should occur 5m before the end of the changeover zone, and because of this each athlete has to sprint more than 100m: the first athlete 105m, the second and third athletes 125m, and the fourth athlete 120m (see Fig. 5.7).

The running position in the lane and the baton exchange for each member of the relay team is as follows:

- The first runner carries the baton in the right hand and runs on the inside of the lane
- The second runner takes the baton in the left hand and runs closer to the outside of the lane
- The third runner takes the baton in the right hand and runs close to the inside of the lane
- The fourth runner takes the baton in the left hand

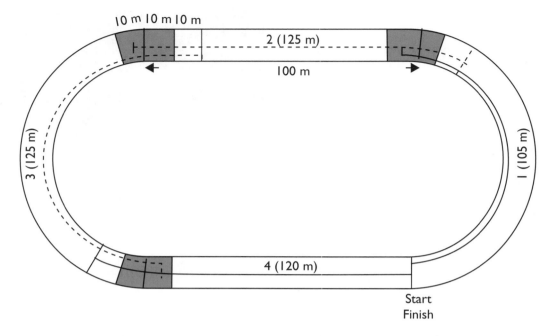

Fig. 5.7: The four legs of the 4 × 100m sprint. Adopted from Mackenzie, B. (2001) *Sprint Relay* **(available from http://www.brianmac.co.uk/sprints/relay.htm).**

The exchange is 'non visual'. Once the outgoing athlete has seen the incoming athlete reach the checkmark, he/she will start as if reacting to the starting gun in a sprint race. The incoming athlete will call 'Hand' when he/she is in a position to pass the baton safely to the outgoing athlete. The outgoing athlete puts back his/her hand, the incoming athlete places the baton into the hand, and the exchange is complete. The outgoing athlete does not watch the baton into his/her hand, hence 'non visual'.

Passing Techniques

There are three common techniques for the athletes to use, depending on their abilities: the upsweep, the downsweep and the push-pass technique.

THE UPSWEEP

In the upsweep the receiving hand is extended behind the athlete at hip height with the palm facing down and a wide angle between the thumb and the rest of the fingers (see Fig. 5.8). The incoming athlete passes the baton in an upward movement into the receiving hand. The advantage of this method is that this is a normal position for the receiving hand. The disadvantage is that it may require some manipulation of the baton in the hand to make the exchange safely.

THE DOWNSWEEP

In the downsweep the receiving hand is extended behind the runner at hip height with the palm facing up and a wide angle between the thumb and the rest of the fingers (see Fig. 5.9). The incoming athlete passes the baton in a downward movement into the receiving hand. The advantage of this method is that

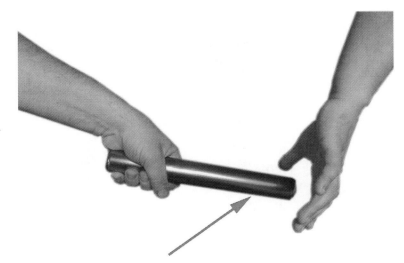

**Fig. 5.8: The upsweep.
(Photo: Geoff Platt)**

it will require no manipulation of the baton to make the next baton exchange safely. A disadvantage is that it is not a natural position for the outgoing athlete's hand to receive the baton.

THE PUSH-PASS TECHNIQUE

In the push-pass technique the outgoing runner's arm is extended out behind them parallel to the ground, and the hand is open with the thumb pointing down (*see* Fig. 5.10). The incoming runner holds the baton vertically and pushes it straight into the open hand.

The advantage of this technique is that the incoming runner can easily adjust the baton's position up, down or sideways, and can observe the outgoing runner's hand take hold of the baton. Also, it will require no manipulation of the baton by the outgoing runner to make the next baton exchange safely. A disadvantage is that it is not a natural position for the outgoing athlete's arm and hand to receive the baton. Nevertheless this is perhaps the safest method of baton exchange.

Selection of Team Members

The performance in the relay event primarily depends upon the perfection of the baton exchange and the sprinting ability of the team. In order to select athletes for the different relay legs it is sensible to find out their capacities

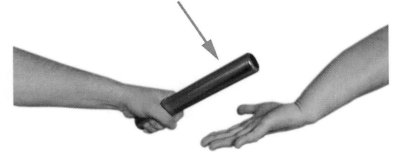

**Fig. 5.9: The downsweep.
(Photo: Geoff Platt)**

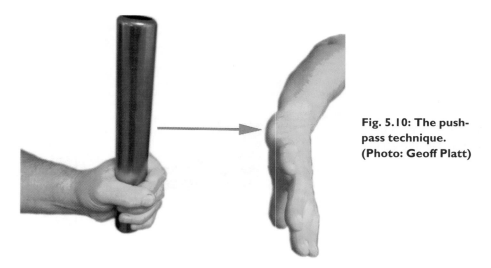

Fig. 5.10: The push-pass technique. (Photo: Geoff Platt)

for a particular section (the second and third runner cover longer distances). It is also advisable to establish each athlete's full potential for running sections on the straight and round the bend. These individual abilities must be taken into account in deciding the running order of a relay team, considering the following:

- First leg: priority goes to an athlete who has a good start, can run the bend, and can pass the baton well
- Second leg: the choice goes to an athlete who is confident in receiving and passing the baton, runs well in the straight, and possesses sufficient speed endurance. The athlete should perhaps be a 200m specialist
- Third leg: the selection goes to the sprinter who is confident and reliable in receiving and passing the baton, can run the bend well, and possesses sufficient speed endurance. The athlete should perhaps be a 200m specialist
- Fourth leg: here we normally select a runner who receives the baton well, is efficient in running the straight, and has a high degree of competitive spirit

CHAPTER 6

PERFORMANCE ANALYSIS IN SPRINTING

by Dr Mohsen Shafizadeh

Performance analysis has been defined as 'An objective way of recording performance, so that critical events can be quantified in a consistent and reliable manner' (Hughes and Bartlett, 2008). It involves the collection of evidence relating to a sports performance in order to assess that performance, and to identify its areas of strength and weakness in order to improve it. Gathering evidence also permits the coach to assert his or her conclusions despite all challenges from the athlete.

Ownership of the data rests with the coach, who must decide how it can be best used in the interests of the athlete. The coach must decide what information should be passed to the athlete, what information should be concealed from them, and whether it is necessary to provide misleading information to them in order to gain an advantage.

'Less is more' is a phrase we use to describe the fact that the functionality of less information is sometimes the same as too much. In addition it represents how important it is for coaches to manage the amount of augmented information that is necessary for performance enhancement. If you have experience of coaching at any level in your preferred sport you have to realize that the main part of your coaching is to provide information to

your athletes in order to correct technique, tactics and strategy. These chunks of information are the result of observation and analysis processes that are *per se* important parts of the coach's duties.

PERFORMANCE ANALYSIS IN MODERN SPORT

Performance analysis and assessment play a significant role in modern sport for a variety of reasons. Firstly, identifying the cause of any performance problem requires precise measurement and evaluation over time (Hughes and Franks, 2008). The feedback-loop process requires the best available data in order to assist the athlete to correct errors and to improve. Unfortunately, accurate feedback is capable of destroying an athlete's self-confidence and self-efficacy, so the coach has a responsibility not to pass it on and either to conceal it, or to supply inaccurate information to the athlete.

Secondly, there are many intervention programmes that are designed by coaches to help athletes. However, if these intervention programmes rely on personal judgment rather than on evidence produced by assessment tools, then the appropriateness of the suggested intervention may be questioned. Performance analysis is defined as an objective way to quantify performance (Hughes and Franks, 2008), and this objectivity is an important part of the decision-making process. In a study conducted in association football it was reported that coaches can recall between 40–45 per cent of events that occur in a match (Laird and Waters, 2008).

Thirdly, performance changes are achieved in the light of continuous development.

In order to monitor performance changes over time (for example daily, weekly, annually) the collection of data on a time basis is crucial. Data management and performance tracking are the main functions of performance analysis in business generally and in sport specifically. Lastly, results from assessment not only provide information to coaches for designing interventions, but also help to scout talented athletes by comparing their performance using a norm-based database.

Another feature of performance analysis that has not been studied extensively is the impact of data, and pundit commentary based on that data, broadcast by the media following major sporting events, and its effect on fans, athletes and coaches. In fact, the television coverage of major events across all sports would be improved if it were accompanied by live, augmented data supported by graphics, charts, maps and drawing tools. A large part of the discussion by panels of expert pundits on television before, during and after an event is related to the interpretation of performance data for viewers. This type of information dissemination has massively influenced the market for user-friendly apps for smartphones and iPads, such as Stats Zone (Opta) and Easy Tag (Dartfish), which replicate the software used in educational and professional sport settings.

This chapter will address the application of performance analysis and performance analysis software in sprinting. The first part of the chapter will reflect on the level of analysis in sport performance generally and on sprint events specifically. In the second part, the methods of feedback provision will be discussed in more detail. As improving performance is the primary aim of the coaching process, providing feedback will be critical due to its guiding role.

THE IMPORTANCE OF COORDINATION

Coordination is an important element of whole body movement in running. Coordination between different limbs is a way to quantify the movement pattern. It is the degree of relationship (or coupling) between joints (limbs) during the execution of a motor skill. For example, during running, the hips, knees and ankles in the lower part of the body and the head, trunk and arms in the upper part of the body move simultaneously to produce a fluent and economic motor skill with minimum energy expenditure (Burkett, 2004).

Generally, there are two types of coordination pattern in any motor skill: inter-limb (between limbs), and intra-limb (within limbs). The coordination between knee and hip of the right leg is an example of intra-limb coordination, whereas the coordination between the right and left hips is an example of inter-limb coordination. The degrees of coordination may be determined by the range of motion and through the relative phase (Stergiou, 2004).

If two limbs move in the same direction the coordination between them is in-phase, such as the contra-lateral motions of the right hand and the left leg during running, and if two limbs move in opposite directions, such as the right hand and the right leg motions, the coordination pattern is anti-phase. Understanding the coordination pattern is necessary in terms of skill acquisition and refinement. In fact, the main part of coach instruction and feedback to novice and expert runners is about how to coordinate different body parts so that the speed of the body is increased.

Gittoes and Wilson (2010), in a study of college sprinters, examined the intra-limb coordination pattern whilst sprinting at maximal speed in a 110m event. They showed that the coupling between knee and ankle (mean RP: 89.9 degrees) was more anti-phase and with less variability compared to the hip-knee coupling (mean RP: 34.2 degrees) across the step phase. On the other hand, in the touchdown the variability between joint couplings was more.

Tom McNab has questioned the value of this type of data to coaches and athletes in his chapter in this book. He points out that whilst collecting such data is useful for producing research papers at university, the very expensive digital camera equipment required in order to measure the joint angles is seldom available to athletes and coaches. In order to use this data the coach would have to find a way to adjust the athlete's joint angle from 95 or 85 degrees to 90 degrees, and the precision necessary to then adjust it from 90 to 89.9 degrees would be unthinkable.

The amount of variability between participants in the touchdown phase is very important for running in maximal velocity, as it allows the runner to transit from the swing to stance through destabilization in the lower-extremity coordination pattern. The more consistent knee-ankle coupling motion suggested that a well trained, healthy sprinter performing in a predictable environment uses a more reproducible knee-ankle coupling motion. Thus, coaching feedback should be selected according to the real nature of the coordination pattern between joints.

Another benefit of variability in the coordination pattern of sprinters is related to the prevention of injury due to overuse syndrome. Patellofemoral pain syndrome (PFP) is the most common running injury, affecting one in four people in the general population, with an even higher incidence among athletes (Barton, Munteanu, Menz and Crossley, 2010; Thijs, De Clercq, Roosen and Witvrouw, 2008). The risk of overuse running injury may not be related to just one mechanism, but rather to the coordination of ankle-knee and hip-knee motions during running, and the variability of that coordination.

The coordination pattern considered to be most relevant to running injuries is the coupling of rear foot eversion, tibial internal rotation and knee flexion (Tiberio, 1987). Some studies reported the reduced variability for injured runners with PFP (Hamill, van Emmerik, Heiderscheit, and Li, 1999). Another factor for the incidence of PFP in runners is duration. Runners with PFP often do not have pain at the beginning of a run, but complain of a gradual onset of pain as the run progresses. This may indicate that running in an exerted state could cause changes in joint coordination or variability which contribute to running injuries such as PFP (Dierks, Manal, Hamill and Davis, 2011). These factors are important training elements for coaches who design repetitive running drills with maximum speed to reach the fatigue threshold.

TACTICAL ANALYSIS FOR SPRINTERS

Races at 100m and 200m for adult athletes are run flat out from gun to tape. However, the lactate threshold means that it is impossible to run flat out for more than 30sec, so 400m runners do need to slow down at some stage of the race in order to complete the distance. If the athlete runs flat out from the gun, then he or she is likely to 'hit the wall' at around 300m so they feel they are 'treading water' and struggling to reach the finishing line, as their rivals, who conserved their energy during the early stages of the race, come bounding past them.

400m running could be continuously changed in terms of pace. From this point of view, understanding the tactics and strategy required to manage the level of energy expenditure is very important for producing an economical movement pattern in the course of competition. So, the next part of this chapter will investigate the time-motion analysis and tactical understanding which is mostly applicable for pacing strategy for 400m sprinters. Technologies are an integral part of performance analysis. As we move from manual and paper-pencil methods of analysis, our dependency on sophisticated systems is increased.

The last section will review the practicality of information technologies in the performance analysis of sprint events.

TECHNICAL ANALYSIS FOR SPRINTERS

The analysis of skills and performance in sprinting may be carried out at both technical and tactical levels. At the technical level, the aim of the analysis is to assess the coordination between the lower extremities to assess technique, so as to refine the athlete's movement pattern and enhance their performance. This level of analysis focuses on the kinematics and kinetics of motion in practice. The technical analysis of running is broadly used by biomechanists and coaches to improve speed or velocity.

Tactics and Strategy

Tactics and strategy are important components of sport and important elements of decision-making. The importance of making a correct decision in many sports has been scientifically studied, but little information exists for sports that require the cyclic, repetitive and continuous execution of a single movement pattern, such as running, swimming and cycling. There are two areas for the application of tactical elements in sprint events: sprinters use a strategy to start the race, and a pacing strategy to maintain maximum speed throughout the entire race. The pacing strategy depends on the duration of the event, with races lasting 30sec or less being run flat out, and those that last more than 30sec requiring the athlete and coach to consider pacing in order to meet the energy requirements of the race.

The strategy of the start relies on the runner's reaction time (RT) and the functioning of the information-processing mechanism in the brain, and to further understand the RT in a sprinter it is helpful to acquire an insight into the different stages of this mechanism. There are three stages in converting a stimulus into a response (Schmidt and Lee, 2011). The first stage is stimulus identification (SI), during which a sprinter picks up information about the sound of the gun. Before the gun is fired to start a race, the starter gives the athletes a 'set' command to prepare them for the sound of the gun. This paradigm is a type of simple RT in which the sprinter is required to respond to only one stimulus at a time. Of course, elite athletes continually practise this vital stage of their event until it becomes automatic and they do not have to waste time considering what to do.

This familiarity with the stimulus in terms of its nature and timing (that is, the time delay between the 'set' command and the gunshot) is an advantage for sprinters who have extensive experience in competitive situations or who know the official starting strategy. According to Collet (1999), most world-class sprinters try to anticipate the starting pistol.

The second stage is response selection (RS). During this stage the sprinter uses working memory to search for appropriate motor programmes in response to a stimulus. In fact, for sprinters who have been exposed to similar situations, it is not difficult to find a solution and send it as a motor command to the limbs for them to start the race.

This stage and the later stage are very time-consuming, and a great portion of RT is spent in the RS and response-planning (RP) stages. The RP stage is the last function of the brain in its preparing for a response. In this stage, all aspects of a correct response, such as the appropriate amount of force, the range of motion and the velocity, are finalized so that the whole package of information is run without any changes. A quicker RT can usually help a sprinter to begin his race properly.

During the 100m sprint, world-class runners spend ~50–60 per cent of the race in the acceleration phase (Tibshirani, 1997). Consequently, 20–25 per cent of the overall work demand of a 100m sprint may be required merely to overcome inertia and alter the body's kinetic energy from rest. Despite the adoption of this all-out strategy, the significant percentage of time spent in the acceleration phase (at low relative speeds) during short sprint events often results in 'negative split' performance times, in which the second half of the race is slower than the first half (van Ingen Schenau et al., 1992; de Koning et al., 1999).

Research has shown that there is a large variation in stride frequency and length among elite sprinters (Salo et al., 2011). Since the athlete's running speed depends on their technique, coaches could well intervene on a practical level to refine the athlete's movement pattern and limb function so as to change their stride length and frequency in order to enhance their performance.

How is Pace Controlled during a 400m Sprint?

The self-selection of exercise intensity may be controlled in a 'teleoanticipatory' manner (Ulmer, 1996), whereby athletes anticipate the work required to complete a given exercise task. St Clair Gibson et al. (2006) have since expanded upon this theory, suggesting that self-selected exercise intensity may be regulated continuously within the brain, based on a complex algorithm involving peripheral sensory feedback and the anticipated workload remaining. It appears that physiological changes within the muscle itself (that is, peripheral fatigue) are also responsible for reductions in power output and subsequent variations in pacing strategies during short- and middle-distance events (Hettinga et al., 2006).

The application of performance analysis for pacing strategy in sprint events, especially in longer distances, would be by the assessment of stride length and cadence over a specific time (for example 2 seconds) or distance (for example 10m) intervals, and by providing feedback to find the best pacing strategy in the course of race. Information regarding acceleration, deceleration and the maintenance phases of a race will help athletes and coaches to plan conditioning programmes according to individual needs.

Environmental conditions can also affect sprinting performance. This has been acknowledged by the IAAF, who measure the wind speed in every competitive race and who refuse to recognize world records set where there is a tailwind of 2.0m.s^{-1}, and advise their constituent members to do the same.

In fact, windy conditions could delay the sprinter achieving maximum velocity, and its effect varies between headwind and tailwind (Linthorne, 1994). Sprinters usually change their tactics in windy conditions by adjusting their body's upright position. Quinn (2010) reported that the most favourable wind condition for sprinters is a wind speed of no more than 2 m.s^{-1}.

Hurdlers dislike *any* wind because their foot placing is exceptionally important to them and a wind will make it impossible to judge that accurately. Rain, sleet and snow will affect body temperature as well as grip of the track. Altitude also affects performance.

TIME-MOTION ANALYSIS IN 400M RACES

One invaluable performance analysis method to understand pacing strategy in 400m sprinters is time-motion analysis. This is a type of qualitative movement analysis model in an actual field in which a whole event could be broken down into small parts according to locomotor movement patterns such as walking, jogging, running and sprinting (O'Donoghue, 2008).

In continuous and cyclic sports such as sprinting, because only one class of movement is used in the entire competition, and only the distance and time are changed, dividing the whole race into reasonable time or distance windows could provide useful information not only for coaches but also for conditioning coaches in terms of physical and physiological preparation. So the 30m sprint time will reflect efficiency out of the blocks, and the 60m sprint time will reflect overall acceleration performance.

For example, the method employed by Bruggerman *et al.* (1999) in the World Athletic Championships in 1997 in Athens in the 100m event was breaking down the event into 10m sections and computing the mean acceleration between successive 10m sections. They reported that the 100m event was comprised of an 'acceleration phase' and a 'peak velocity phase'.

Korhonen *et al.* (2003) used the same method of time-motion analysis, but calculated other parameters in 10m-distance sections such as stride length, stride rate, ground contact time and flight time during the acceleration, peak velocity and deceleration phases. However, the main purpose of this study was the comparison of 100m performance between different age groups (forty to ninety years) – but the method of movement classification is applicable to elite and non-elite sprinters in different events in order to provide knowledge about sprinters' strategy in control of the pace. In addition, split times can be compared between different groups of athletes in terms of age, level of expertise and experience, and gender in order to provide a better insight into an individualized training plan and areas for improvement.

FEEDBACK PROVISIONS AND INFORMATION TECHNOLOGY

Coaching science informs us that the coach's first responsibilities after a race include providing positive feedback to the athlete in order to reaffirm his or her self-confidence and self-efficacy. The next priorities include a possible lap of honour, as well as the requirements of the Press and the anti-drug testers. The athlete's need to re-hydrate and re-energize should also be addressed. Only when these tasks have been completed can the coach consider delivering serious feedback to the athlete.

Initial skill acquisition and refinement requires a step-by-step process in which relevant information is presented in stages, according to the phases of learning. For example, the important information that is provided during the presentation of a new skill is through instruction and demonstration. Thus a coach verbally informs the learners about the correct technique, and then demonstrates it in order to give a visual picture of the movement pattern. The importance of explicit methods in learning motor skills is discussed in more detail in previous studies (see Hodges and Williams, 2012).

Following practice, athletes need to receive feedback on their performance. Augmented feedback is defined as any external source of information to help an athlete regarding the quality and outcome of his performance (Schmidt and Lee, 2011). It may be presented personally or through machines such as computers, although allowing the athlete direct access to data prevents any manipulation of that data, and giving him access to a computer sets a precedent that cannot then be broken when things go wrong and the data causes the athlete to have a nervous breakdown in the middle of an Olympic final.

For example, when a sprinter finishes a 100m race, he/she needs feedback about the outcome of the race in terms of time. Usually a stopwatch is the tool selected to provide the feedback. This type of feedback, relating to the results of a race, is called 'knowledge of results' (KR). KR is helpful for events that require objective assessment in terms of time, distance, score and so on.

However, the quality of a skill is not improved by KR. Knowledge of performance (KP) is another type of feedback that informs a runner about the quality of technique. Many aspects of coaching for sprinters focus on the

ways to improve running mechanics and the efficiency of technique. Thus, in each training session coaches usually provide verbal comments aimed at refining a movement pattern. A combination of KP and KR is very useful in coaching sprinters because it focuses on both technique and results.

One important feature of KP is the method employed to present the feedback to the athlete. There are two ways to present KP: descriptive and prescriptive. Frequently, providing KP regarding the quality of past performance is neither informative nor sufficient to refine the skill. For example, 'your knees were bent at take-off' is a coaching comment that describes the performance only in terms of correct and wrong qualities. Another way to present this verbal KP is by prescribing a solution to change it: for example, 'during take-off, push your body up and forwards'. If a novice performer has different solutions for each problem, then gradually the problem-solving ability will be expanded during the athlete's development process.

Technology using video feedback has been widely used in modern sport over recent decades. In fact, many coaches rely on video feedback in their training sessions in order to improve performance in different levels of performers (for example, novices and experts). Depending on the available technology, the provision of video KP may be simple or complex. For example, using a handycam for recording and replaying the movement is a simple way to present KP. Because the performance is recorded and stored in hardware (such as a camera or personal computers), reviewing performance is possible at any time, but this method cannot provide much information about the quality of technique.

Nowadays, sophisticated software packages are used by coaches and analysts to provide feedbacks. For example, Dartfish (Dartfish Co.) has introduced different products for performance analysis of individual and team sports. The advantage of this system for an analyst is in the recording and analysing of an event through live or recorded options by connecting to a digital camera and using analyser options in the software to provide different kinds of feedback immediately after completing a skill. In addition, it is possible to compare different performances by split screens, and to highlight the strengths and weaknesses of the performance by drawing tools. These functions in software could facilitate the movement evaluation because they show the performance errors and also the coaches' comments on a video clip.

Understanding pacing strategy is another characteristic of information technology and video feedbacks. For example, if the purpose of analysis is to understand the different phases of a sprint race in terms of acceleration, maintenance and deceleration, then breaking down the race into 10m distances and presenting the spent time in each time slot is a preferred method of feedback.

CONCLUSION

Performance analysis is a system of recording and analysing athlete performance using staff and equipment outside the usual athlete/coach team, so that it may be evaluated against the performance of other, better athletes or the previous performances of the same athlete. The data is accurate and objective, and it belongs to the coach.

Interpretation of the data, and the intelligent use of it, is the responsibility of the coach, who will employ his knowledge, skills and experience to know what and how to best advise the athlete in the heat of competition in order to secure the best possible results achievable by the athlete on the day.

CHAPTER 7

COACHING SPRINTING

An Interview with Tom McNab

Q. Do you have any general coaching principles?
A. To do only what is necessary, rather than what is possible, and to make it specific. Much of what now comes to us from the top derives from coaches working with full-time athletes, much of it irrelevant to the contexts within which most of our coaches work.

Q. Which are?
A. Basic teaching to the ten-to-thirteen age group, the coaching of committed teenagers in the fourteen-to-eighteen territory, then the coaching of committed senior athletes. The first group has narrow technical parameters, and is essentially an education, a set of lessons with a strong five-star element. That means a high emphasis on timing and measuring, because this will be the only opportunity in a lifetime for these children to experience competitive athletics.

The second group (fourteen to eighteen) is almost invariably in groups, and if it is within a club, it is rarely with a high quality specialist coach. Even outside a club, with a specialist coach, it is often in large groups, and the same is true in the senior group; this is the product of a diminishing stock of coaches.

Q. So one-to-one coaching is relatively rare?
A. Yes, in the sense of what occurred with Harry Wilson and Steve Ovett, and Seb Coe and his dad. What I am about to discuss is the product of one-to-one coaching, but I will try to fillet out what can be deployed in a group situation.

Q. And your next principle?
A. Keep it simple! Einstein said that any fool could make things complicated, but it took a genius to simplify them. Reduce everything to simple basics. I have recently read massive tomes on sprinting which I have found it impossible to understand, all about shin angles and the like. Now I am certain that these works are, in sports science terms, impeccable, but they are of little practical use. Sports science is a muddy river which must always be carefully filtered.

Q. But it should surely act as our guide?
A. Yes. But it should inform rather than direct. No sports scientist in history ever invented a technique or training method: those were always created by coaches and athletes. No, it must inform coaching, rather than lead it. The problem is that making things complicated always pays better. The great American coach Lawson Robertson once observed that

if a coach came to you with complex training systems you could be sure of only one thing – that he was trying to sell you something.

Thus in recent years we have been engulfed in a welter of drills and exercises. But if we look at what has happened here (particularly in women's athletics), we see that for all of the science, our women now rank in the 100/200 well below what they did thirty years ago. This is something that has no parallel in any other British sport. We have had several girls who have run in the mid-elevens at age fifteen (about two seconds faster than Andrea Lynch did at the same age), but whose eventual senior world rankings were about fifty places lower. Full-time athletics and sports science didn't do much for them. Reality is a bitch.

Q. What was your first experience of coaching?
A. Coaching myself in triple jump, because back in Scotland in the 1950s there was no coaching of field events. I had to make some crude analysis of the event, and then try in practice to 'read' what I was doing. So I have always had sympathy for people who seemed to lack natural talent (I wasn't even the best athlete in my street!), and have always tried to break down events into easily learned chunks. At the age of twenty-six I had cleared 14.91 in triple jump, and by the time I was thirty I'd won five Scottish titles.

Q. And coaching athletes?
A. The first was by accident, and it may be worth describing it, if only to give hope to novice coaches. I was still a competitive athlete back in 1957 when I convinced my club, Shettleston Harriers, to buy pole-vault equipment. A fortnight later my club sec-retary, Davie Ferguson, asked me where all the vaulters were, as if they would suddenly spring from the earth simply because he had provided the equipment. I looked across

the track, identified a skinny fifteen-year-old, Norrie Foster, and called him over.

I had read in a Webster book about the Birkett exercise, where the coach holds the pole and swings the novice over. I dragged Norrie over about two metres on that first session, and in the following weeks moved on to short-run vaults with support, then vaults on his own. That year he won the Scottish Schools title, and four years later the British Junior title. I then moved him on to decathlon and a British title, and he was fourth in both events at the 1966 Commonwealth Games in Jamaica.

Q. Lesson?
A. If you wait until you know all about the mechanics of an event, you will end up an old man, and as a result lots of young athletes will have missed out.

Q. When did you first start coaching sprints?
A. Back in 1963, when I was first appointed National Coach. The moment you secure an official position, everyone immediately assumes that you know something. And so it was for me back then – athletes immediately asked me to coach them, though I had little coaching experience.

Fortunately for me, one of my first was Madeleine Cobb, a tough, strong-willed, national-level sprinter who had just had a baby. She was at that point understandably unfit and overweight, and capable of around 13.0sec for 100m with the wind behind her and her mother on the stop-watch.

Q. So what did you do?
A. I immediately contacted a colleague, Bill Marlow, who had taken Peter Radford to a world 200m record and an Olympic bronze in 100m in Rome. Bill was a pragmatic coach of the old school, strong on good running tech-nique, and on always working at the 90–100

per cent level. He provided me with some simple bread-and-butter practices, which I immediately applied.

Q. And the result?
A. Madeleine ran 11.5 and 23.6 on cinders, winning several British indoor titles and a silver in the relay at the Commonwealth Games in 1970.

Q. Were you working at the same time on other events?
A. Yes – in triple jump with Fred Alsop, who got fourth in the Tokyo Olympics in 1964. I always reckoned that if I had been more experienced, then Fred would certainly have medalled. But experience is something you get about fifteen minutes after you needed it.

This being said, Fred had never even won a national title up to that point, and his 16.65w on the harsh White City cinders is a distance that none of our present jumpers can guarantee.

Q. So what had you learnt?
A. That you learn from experience. I drew on Bill Marlow's experience in my work with Cobb, and from my own in triple jump in coaching Alsop. And with those two experiences with tough, committed athletes, I had also learnt a lot from them. And I have always been a compulsive reader. I was slowly educating myself as a coach.

Q. Your next sprinter?
A. Paradoxically, a twenty-six-year-old sailor, Peter Gabbett, who came to me for decathlon in 1966, with only 11.0 for 100m and around 52sec for 400m. Speed is vital in decathlon, it runs through it like the veins through the body, so with Peter I applied an enhanced version of the practices that I had developed with Madeleine Cobb. It was still simple stuff.

Q. And what did Gabbett end up with?
A. 10.3 and 46.10, at age thirty-two, the latter standing for many years as the best ground-level 400m ever run in decathlon. And a score of 8,040 points, the first British athlete to go beyond 8,000 points.

Q. Who was your next sprinter?
A. Andrea Lynch in 1968, a seventeen-year-old, with bests of around 12.5/26.0. In 1969 she gained silver at the European Juniors, and in 1974 a 100m silver at the Commonwealth and gold in the 60m European Indoors. But her greatest achievement was to rank number two in the Track and Field News world rankings in 1973. This is the highest ranking ever achieved in 100m by a British woman.

Q. But we have had girls as much as a second faster at fifteen than Andrea was at seventeen, but who never went anywhere close to that ranking.

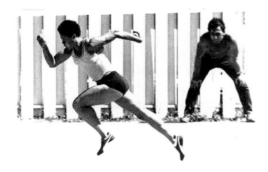

Fig. 7.1: Tom McNab coaching Andrea Lynch at Crystal Palace in 1975.

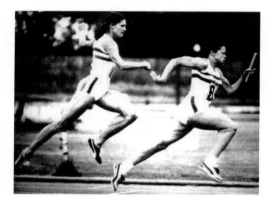

Fig. 7.2: Judy Vernon hands over to Andrea Lynch in the Great Britain versus German Democratic Republic match at Crystal Palace in 1975.

A. Yes, much better material, at least in the physical sense. But what you can't tell is what level of mental strength these girls possessed, or their capacity to take training. This being said, some of them must have had it, but nothing much seems to have happened. My guess is that they simply weren't exposed to an environment that would take them to world class.

Q. Did anyone ever ask you what you had done with Andrea?
A. No, not a single coach, and this may tell you something about British coaching culture. Similarly, many years later no one ever asked how in two years Greg Rutherford went from being a footballer who had never won a county title to being a world-class sprinter/jumper. And not a single question either from anyone in the governing body.

Q. But coaching isn't always easy to explain, beyond describing training sessions.
A. Yes, what is always hard to explain is the intensity, the passion of the sessions, the quality of focus. And equally difficult to describe are the off-track informal discussions, phone calls, the post-race analysis, stuff like that. That's why much of coach education tends to be reduced to formulae, to recipes, to coaching as simply a collection of drills and exercises, detached from practice.

Q. I hear that the coaches of our funded athletes now have to submit their programmes to a head-office coach for scrutiny.
A. Madness – there's no way anyone can make such assessments. And the fact that they think they can only makes me question their knowledge of coaching. Again, it aims to reduce coaching to sets of recipes. Now, this is not an argument against training programmes, only one against detailed forward plans, indeed anything much beyond describing general training priorities and competitive aims. Because much of coaching has to be done on the balls of the feet.

Q. Is it the same with much of our sports science?
A. In some ways, yes. Coaching must always have a rational base from which to operate, and it provides that base, but the danger is always unfiltered sports science. By that I mean information which has not passed through the sieve of practical experience, which has not been, in effect, pre-digested.

Q. Meaning to separate the wheat from the chaff, to establish the priorities?
A. Exactly. In the past we had coaches like Dyson and Paish, men with a PE background and considerable coaching experience, who would filter sports science before

they delivered its product to coach education. That is no longer so. And so we have on the one hand foreign coaches delivering complex and irrelevant drills and exercises, and on the other sports scientists dumping unfiltered training theory. All science is provisional, and training theory is just that – theory.

Q. But surely Dyson was one of the fathers of sports science?

A. Yes, but Dyson understood its relevance, he knew where it should be placed. I remember him telling me that he would often meet coaches who could discuss the mechanics of an event with him in great detail, but who had never coached. To him, such 'coaches' were simply irrelevant.

Q. Has this mix of foreign coaches and unadulterated sports science had malign effects on sprints coaching?

A. Yes. Probably more than on field events, where most of our coaching is being done by ex-athletes who have a pretty good idea of what their event is about. As a consequence, sprints coaching has been smothered in a welter of drills and exercises. Thus we see athletes walking backwards, ducking under and over hurdles, repetition crawling, shuttle running at jogging speeds, the list is endless. We are seeing something more akin to the work of a health-club instructor than a coach, a random collection of exercises delivered to athletes, regardless of age. This is recipe coaching, compounded by the fact that groups are getting larger, taking us even further away from one-to-one coaching.

Q. The loss of the personal touch?

A. Yes. So everyone in the group does everything. The problem is that young sprinters almost inevitably get better simply by working with other sprinters, maturing, getting experience of competition. The coach naturally thinks that this improvement is the product of his junk exercise, and who would attempt to argue with him, who indeed can prove otherwise? I improved from 12.2 to 11.5 from age eighteen to age twenty-seven, without a moment's coaching, indeed without even training with other athletes. Now, I would not recommend this to anyone, but it shows what can be done without coaching, indeed without indoor training facilities and with limited competition. Had a coach been involved, then he would undoubtedly have claimed the credit.

Q. Can a sprints coach 'get off' with much more than, say, a pole-vault coach?

A. Yes, there is no doubt about it. Rafilli took Holly Bleasdale from zero at age sixteen in vault to 4.87m at age twenty. A sprinter like Gemilli came out of football with only a few months training and ran 10.06, a performance of similar calibre. Top sprinters sometimes come to the event at sixteen/seventeen, often within 4 per cent of their ultimate best time, which is a totally different situation as compared to the coach in a technical event like pole vault, which develops, quite literally, from the ground up.

Q. But isn't there a danger that we become too inward-looking?

A. That's true, but we have shown a costly naiveté in our search for a Wizard of Oz. Thus foreign coaches have arrived with us with tenuous connections with great athletes, or others who, in the American college system, have been able to work with superb talent. And we have believed that what they tell us can be directly applied to athletes in quite different club situations. Millions have been spent in appointing these wizards, who have departed these shores considerably richer, but leaving little more behind them than a pottage of drills and exercises.

Q. What impact has this had upon coach education?

A. Coach education has been reduced to performance by powerpoint, plus a disconnected collection of articles and lectures on the web. Now much of what is delivered is probably, in sports science terms, 'correct', but it is rarely of any practical value. And much of the filmed lecture material is desperately amateurish, raw, single camera stuff, when what is required is multi-camera material, professionally edited. This quality of coach education is nothing less than a misuse of public funds.

Getting back to my 'Oz' analogy, remember that when Dorothy finally gets to meet the wizard, she finds that he is only a confused old man fumbling away behind a curtain. The best advice she gets is from Glinda, the good witch: 'There's no place like home.' We have sufficient expertise in this country to meet most of our educational needs, but it is not being effectively deployed.

Q. So it isn't lack of information?

A. No – we are drowning in information, but there is a lack of intelligent selection and practical application of the knowledge that already exists. And there is an unwillingness to ask those who have been consistently successful within our system how they did it.

Q. You mean, to see what can be learnt from them?

A. Exactly. Jim Spooner produced in Kathy Cooke a 22.1 200m runner over thirty years ago, but has a path been beaten to his door to ask him how that was achieved? Or was Cooke simply a freak of nature? I don't think so. This mulish unwillingness to consult with other coaches is one of our central problems. Coaches will pay fortunes to listen to the wizards, but they won't take the trouble to pick up the phone to seek the advice of a successful coach in their own country.

Q. But isn't it true that it isn't always possible to pass on the intensity, the environment that a great coach creates?

A. That is so – that is the ghost in the machine. At best he can only give a hint of it in a lecture or a conversation. The best in literature is probably the American Dean Cromwell in his 1940 book *Championship Track and Field Athletics*, and I suspect that it was his co-author Wesson who managed to give the real flavour of Cromwell's work. In 1948 Dyson and his colleagues visited Cromwell in his London hotel with pencils and empty notebooks. They left three hours later with their notebooks still empty. For Cromwell, for all the great athletes that he had coached, did not speak their language. And his success wasn't simply because he had the cream of the crop at his disposal, it was because of the environment that he created, and the college competitive system. Dyson and his coaches were almost certainly asking the wrong questions, or Cromwell was unable to find the right words, and that was why they left the meeting disappointed. But I remember Cromwell's phrase, 'I call all my boys champ, and some of them believe me': good coaches go far beyond the technical – they create the expectation of success.

Q. OK, so let's look at your own direct experience of sprints coaching.

A. First, let me make it clear that my main work has been done with 100m runners, long jumpers and decathletes. But let me also make it clear that none of the athletes with whom I worked was already an exceptional sprinter: Andrea Lynch at age seventeen, 12.5, Peter Gabbett at age twenty-six, 11.0/52.0, and Greg Rutherford at age sixteen, 11.5 – those were their starting ages and performances. The end result was Lynch at age twenty-three with 10.9, Gabbett at age thirty-two with 10.3/46.1, and Rutherford at age eighteen with 10.38.

And let me also make it clear that I do not suggest that my methods are the only way to coach sprinters, though they may offer up some material which can be interpolated into other systems.

Q. Can you summarize your sprints philosophy?
A. Yes: it is force plus cadence, all glued together by good technique.

Q. What about periodization?
A. There are, to my knowledge, at least three periodization theories: those of Veroshensky, Matveyev and Tschiene. I make no claim to understanding the subtle differences between these contending theories, and I suspect that there will be few who do so. But it is interesting to note that in swimming some coaches have moved away from the long slow base, moving to fast swimming as the season approaches. No, they have started with speed from the outset, increasing in volumes as the season approaches.

There is no need for a big aerobic base for short sprinters, whose VO_2 levels are usually around 60. I now use the hard 30sec run, with 4min rest between runs, starting at 4min, and building to 6min in the October period. This has the advantage of being at decent speed, not far from 80 per cent. Alas, I have seen coaches using 20m shuttle runs at around 19sec 100m speed, which is absolutely pointless.

And all through this period there are always the running practices over 30–50m at around 90 per cent effort, six per set, at least two sets per session, that is, around 500m.

Q. Weights?
A. With Rutherford and Lynch, no. In the case of Rutherford, he only trained for around six hours a week, because of studies. The other reason was a practical one, simply that I could find nowhere local for him to train with weights. I would now deploy a basic strength period from October to December, moving on to a lightweight power period from January to May, then maintenance. But my problem is that I am now coaching teenagers in full-time education, almost all triple jumpers for whom sprints is only part of their programme, so I tend to omit weights.

Q. Stretching?
A. Recent research has shown that slow stretching may actually damage muscle. Any study of ballet dancers would have shown that years ago. My objection to them was always that the exercises did not replicate the actual movements made in the act of running. So I have always used ballistic stretching, deploying movements and movement ranges that simulate running actions. But not many.

Q. Plyometrics?
A. Mainly for cadence, two-footed hurdles bound with toe landings, say, three sets of six per session, or standing spring jumps.

Q. OK, so let's look at the running practices.
A. Fortunately I filmed my first session with Andrea Lynch in 1968, then three further films in the 1968–76 period, one in which she went from an unranked UK athlete to Track and Field News world number two ranking in 1973 and number three in 1974. So there is visual evidence of what happened, quite separate from times and medals. Almost all of Andrea's work was technical, over distances from 30m to 300m.

The first film shows a chunky, low-hipped wee girl of seventeen, with a cross arm action, the second a more muscular creature with a more linear arm action. The third shows her a year or so later, running taller and much more muscular, and the final film (taken at Crystal Palace in the same straight as the 1968 film) shows a lean, high-hipped, fluent runner, now world class. In all films she is the same height and weight. I only took two films of her start and pick-up. The first, in 1968, shows a short, low-range movement, the second, six years later, long, rangy movements from the start through the pick-up.

The point that I wish to make is that there was no magic in any of this, only rep after rep on each practice, hundreds of them, with the muscles gradually making the necessary adaptations. And although this is something that is less easy to put on paper, there was the slow, steady honing of a competitive athlete, dozens of observed races and informal discussions. The soft skills.

Q. You say that your practices were over 30m to 50m, in sets of six, three on each practice?
A. Yes. The first is a jog-in, on toes, with high hips, running in at 90 per cent effort, holding the hips high, with low shoulders and a vertical trunk (see Fig. 7.1). This is the basic sprint shape. Now, no one gets this immediately, but over time they will, or something approximate to it.

Q. And the second?
A. What I call 'lip to hip' in terms of arm action (see Figs 7.1 and 7.2). This is to fix the basic arm action, to make athletes aware of what their arms do: thumbs up, hands slightly inwards, but not across the body. This finishes off the first six reps.

Q. What about open hands?
A. That's fine by me, as long as they are loose. The third practice, beginning the second set of six, often has dramatic effects. It is what I call the 'jelly jaw' practice. The jaw must be loose, and hands and wrists relaxed.

Q. What is the rest between sets?
A. About four minutes, when the athlete can have a drink.

Q. And the second set of three?
A. Elbow drive. This has to be done at close to full speed. Here I stress the drive back of the elbows, keeping the elbow angle steady (see Fig. 7.3).

Q. And to end the set?
A. Usually a test of what has already been covered, by running 50m, with the first 25m at 90 per cent and the second half stressing elbow drive. Here, I watch to see if relaxation is held in that second half.

Q. Are these all of the practices?
A. No. These are the sets that are a sort of bedrock, those that I am happy to introduce even with novice teenage sprinters, rep after rep. And here I would note that it may take some time before all of even these broad technical elements are effectively expressed, moving them up to longer training distances. Now I would like to move on to some of the more complex movements which are further up the food chain, so to speak.

The first is driving practice. This is quite separate from the previous practices, which are from a jog-on start. Its essence is pushing over a full range of movement, through a trunk with head in line. The photograph of Andrea shows her at her very best. We see here a full straight-line drive, but again I must stress that there is no quick fix. This took years of work and began at age seventeen with short, weak drive-out strides.

Q. From blocks?
A. No. The practice is from a standing or three-point start. First, the leg angles, 90 degrees for the front leg, about 120 degrees for the back leg, with the front foot directly under the centre of gravity. The aim is a two-footed drive, but the aim initially is full extension from the front leg.

Here, eye focus is important, with the eyes

focused on the ground where the front foot will strike, and no lifting of the head. The 'feel' is that someone has pinned the back leg to the ground, a long, pushing movement. It is a spring-out at about 45 degrees, similar to a standing long jump, and after a few reps the distance from the front foot to the first contact will increase.

We now ask the athlete to repeat the same 'clinging' movement through the first ten strides, say six reps.

Q. Is all of this flat out?
A. Yes, unlike the earlier running practices, there can be no 90 per cent efforts. And we can insert elbow drive, re-introducing another element in the vocabulary into a different practice.

Q. How does this translate into actual starting?
A. Very easily, for without realizing it your athlete has already being performing starting practices (albeit without blocks) for months. Greg Rutherford had never, till age eighteen, competed in sprints for his club, but he was suddenly asked to do so, with a previous best at age sixteen of around 11.5. I bought him a set of blocks, we put the same driving-practice 'shape' into the blocks, and he ran 10.75 that Saturday after two sessions off blocks. In his next race, at Mannheim, he ran 10.38. All of this was done without weights, without walking around backwards or in slow motion, or ducking under hurdles. Since then, over seven years he has probably more than doubled his training loads, lifted hundreds of tons of weights, and has run $\frac{1}{10}$sec faster.

Q. Can you go into detail about transfer to blocks?
A. Here goes. The American Franklin Henry, way back in the period directly after World War II, conducted experiments on differ-

ent methods of starting, and concluded that the medium start produced the best block velocity. To my knowledge, no research since then has questioned his conclusions, which was essentially a two-footed drive out, with an impulse of around 0.125 off the back foot and around 0.320 off the front foot. But when we look at most sprinters we rarely see any impulse from the back leg.

Q. Which foot should lead?
A. The strongest leg, usually the left. It should be placed directly under the centre of gravity, on a shallow front block, with the weight placed forward, the shoulders directly above the hands, so that when the hips are lifted into the 'set', the sprinter is immediately locked in position.

Q. Front leg angle?
A. Ninety degrees, with the back leg shallow, at around 120 degrees. This means hips above shoulders. The sprinter must go actively into the blocks, 'feeling' them as he goes in, for this is his launch pad.

Q. Eye focus?
A. Down and ahead, with the head in line with the spine. The take of the drive angle is the same as the standing long jump, 45 degrees. If the head comes up on the gun, then the horizontal impulse will be weaker. The aim is a full extension from both legs, 'holding' the block off the front leg, then the same action, stride after stride through the pick-up, basically a repetition of driving practice.

Q. Harness running?
A. Yes, over 20 to 30m.

Q. What other practices?
A. This next one is a wee bit more complex, and I would only deploy it with more advanced athletes. It is over 30 to 50m at 90

per cent full speed, and the active pull-back of the lead thigh is particularly important if the sprinter tends to flick out his lead leg, causing braking.

Q. Any others?

A. There is cadence practice, which is simply a shortening of the arm action at 90–100 per cent effort. Finally there is 'tunnelling', which can be done at any level. That is not technical, but is rather psychological, and involves the blocking out of anything on either side, the feeling of running through a tunnel.

Q. What about over-distance training?

A. Sets of 150s, 200s, 250s, 300s, with long rests between. In every run, the aim must be to keep good form under fatigue, keeping shape, so that this becomes automatic. So we may have four by 200m differential, with the first 100m at 90 per cent effort and the second at 100 per cent, with complete recovery, or two by 300m with the first 100m at 80 per cent, the second at 90 per cent and the third at 100 per cent, again with complete recovery. Constantly vary the effort level, but always with good technique. Going into the season, cut the volume, increase the intensity. But to keep it interesting, the coach should always ring the changes. As an example, driving practice can be spiced up by making it a relay change, with marks out of a hundred for the best changes in the group. Athletes love this 'Strictly Come Dancing' session.

Q. There is no magic to all of this, is there?

A. The Nobel physicist Ralph Feynman said that we learn nothing from science. No, he said, we learn from experience. Anyone can make things difficult, in effect surround athletes in a wilderness of drills and exercises, a sea of irrelevance. What is hard in a discussion like this is to describe the focus, the intensity of good coaching, the environment that the coach creates for his athletes. That is hard to put in words. My Rutherford/Gabbett/Lynch experience is small in numbers, but the record is 100 per cent, all with athletes of no great natural ability.

What I have discussed with you is a short summary of my life in coaching, one in which sprinting has played only a small part. One of the advantages I and the other national coaches of my period had, men like John Anderson and Wilf Paish, was experience of physical education, often in difficult circumstances. We also had experience of a range of events, and even of other sports. All of this was threaded into whatever event that we coached, whatever situation we encountered.

Q. That is now rare.

A. Yes, and it was particularly valuable in training coaches who had to work in schools or in club situations, ones in which they were not working with mature, committed athletes, situations in which athletics has to be vigorously 'sold'. And that is where most coaches now find themselves, rather than in one-to-one situations with full-time senior athletes. And where they are working with smaller groups, with committed teenage athletes, what I describe is even more relevant: how to achieve national and even international levels of performance in no more than five to six hours a week.

Q. Can you summarize your philosophy in a few words?

A. Less is more, so it is always quality rather than quantity, and specificity. And running through every moment is focus on some element of the event.

Q. Have you any final message?

A. Yes. Don't be a chipolata from the coach education machine. The good coach sees exactly what everybody else sees, but does something completely different.

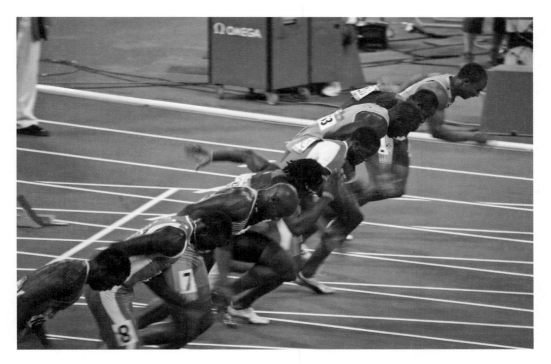

Fig. 7.3: Usain Bolt on his way to a new world record in the 100 metres Olympic final in Beijing, 2008. (Photo: Shutterstock)

CHAPTER 8

TRAINING METHODS 1960–2014

by Dr Geoffrey K. Platt

In order to become a world-class sprinter you must do more than just sprint: you must become bigger, stronger, fitter and faster than you need to be in order to run the world record for your event. If you do not do this then you will be injured when something happens that is just a little more testing than normal, and if this injury occurs shortly before a major event, such as an Olympic final, then you will have wasted years of strenuous effort. Of course, this does not mean that all sprinters need to become weightlifters or supermen.

Since 1960, Great Britain and Northern Ireland have produced some truly outstanding world-class sprinters, men such as Peter Radford, Allan Wells, Cameron Sharp, Mike Macfarlane, Linford Christie, Dwain Chambers, Darren Campbell, Jason Gardener, James Dasoulu, Harry-Aikinees-Areetey and Adam Gemili. Unfortunately our women have not been as successful, with just Dorothy Hyman circuit training.

This chapter will review and evaluate each of the following training methods:

- Speedball
- Plyometrics
- Multigym
- Olympic weightlifting
- Powerlifting

CIRCUIT TRAINING

Circuit training is, as the name suggests, an exercise programme in which a number of exercises, focusing on each part of the body in turn, are undertaken in rotation, with time-limited breaks between each exercise and each circuit. It targets strength building, muscular endurance and fitness. Novices may start with two- or three-minute breaks, but these will normally reduce sharply over a short period. It is generally accepted that R. E. Morgan and G. T. Anderson from the University of Leeds created the concept of circuit training in 1953.

There is one fundamental problem with circuit training, and that is finding and securing the use of suitable equipment. Circuit training requires a school gymnasium equipped with wall bars, benches, medicine balls and mats. Unfortunately, the number of these has become drastically reduced in recent years as the physical education curriculum has changed from gymnastics to games and sports; and the number of schools that hire out their facilities to sports clubs has also been reduced. The equipment takes time to set up and put away, and this effort means that a substantial number of athletes must be available to use the equipment.

The usual exercises for circuit training include the following:

Upper body:
- Squat-ups
- Bench dips
- Back extensions
- Medicine ball chest pass
- Bench lift
- Inclined press-up

Core and trunk:
- Sit-ups (lower abdominals)
- Stomach crunch (upper abdominals)
- Back extension chest raise

Lower body:
- Squat jumps
- Compass jumps
- Astride jumps
- Step-ups
- Shuttle runs
- Hopping shuttles
- Bench squat

Total body:
- Burpees
- Treadmills
- Squat thrusts
- Skipping
- Jogging

Research undertaken by Baylor University and the Cooper Institute has shown that circuit training is the most time-efficient way to enhance cardiovascular fitness and muscle endurance. For example, Peter Radford, the former world record holder for the 200m and the Olympic bronze medallist in the 100m in Rome in 1960, relied on circuit training to support his sprinting.

SPEEDBALL

A speedball is the leather football suspended from the ceiling of a gymnasium that boxers are frequently seen punching, on films and on television, so that it bounces away and then back again, for the boxer to hit again. It assists boxers to improve their endurance, fitness, co-ordination and skill.

In Scotland there is a long history of professional sprinting, including the Powderhall Sprints, which took their name from an area lying between Broughton Road and Warriston Road in the north of Edinburgh, the Scottish capital. Until recently it was best known for Powderhall Stadium, a greyhound racing track, which has now closed. The Sprints, first held in 1870, comprised a series of professional handicap footraces run at the stadium, and which, since 1999, have continued as the 'New Year Sprints', now held at Musselburgh Racecourse.

Credit for introducing the speedball into sprinting goes to Jim Bradley, who was born and brought up close to Powderhall Stadium in a single room tenement in Broughton Street. Seeking ways to support himself after periods of unemployment and in the Army, he became a professional sprinter and then a professional sprint coach. He recognized that sprinters take five strides per minute and that speedball users hit the ball five times per minute, giving them a similar cadence.

The Powderhall sprinters used to train in local boxing gymnasia and came to use the speedballs which, they felt, improved their hand and arm speed, which in turn improved their leg speed. It should, therefore, come as no surprise that when Allan Wells and Cameron Sharp, both from the area, achieved world class in sprinting, they both came to rely on the speedball as part of their training programmes.

The benefits of using a speedball include the following:

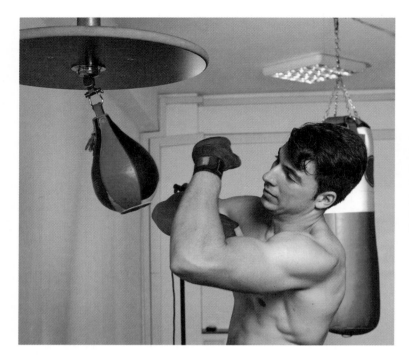

Fig. 8.1: The benefits for the sprinter using a speedball as part of their training programme are well documented. (Photo: Shutterstock)

Improved fitness: Punching the speedball requires the athlete to hold up their arms and hands for extended periods of time, building shoulder and arm strength, as well as endurance. Punching repeatedly for a period of time, such as three minutes, also has cardiovascular benefits. With training, this can be extended to fifteen minutes or longer, helping to increase aerobic capacity. Moving around the platform and introducing other movements such as marching whilst doing so, further benefits the legs.

Confidence: Sprinters have to learn how to hit the speedball (or bag). It takes time, effort and concentration to do it well, and athletes are often frustrated when they start trying to hit it. However, when they start to get their rhythm and learn how to do it, they will start to improve very quickly. And as they improve their quickness, hand speed and eye–hand coordination, their confidence

grows, and that also helps their sprint performance.

Eye–hand co-ordination: Hitting a speedball with single or multiple punches, using one or both hands, requires continuous work, consistency and timing. The athlete can do this standing relatively still, facing the bag, or by moving around the bag, with basic footwork, so that hitting and moving become second nature.

Rhythm and timing: By maintaining a constant and continuous speedball motion using both hands and arms with equal force and speed the athlete will improve their rhythm and timing.

Hand speed and punching power: Keeping the speedball moving at a constant speed requires equal punching power and hand speed. As hand speed increases, so does the power of the punching. Increasing the hand speed also helps to eliminate wasted motion and to improve accuracy.

Speedballs are popular with both genders and all ages, as well as athletes with a disability. They allow athletes to work inside in poor weather conditions, and are seen almost as toys, despite encouraging strenuous exercise. Speedballs do, however, have to be adjusted to the athlete, so that the weight and height of the ball, and the resistance of the swivel, are all adjusted to suit the individual. Athletes also need to wear a good pair of gloves in order to protect themselves from injury.

PLYOMETRICS

Plyometrics is defined as 'a form of training that develops explosive power. It consists of performing hops, bounds and jumps so that maximum effort is expended while a muscle group is lengthening. During plyometrics, a concentric muscle action (shortening) is immediately followed by an eccentric action (lengthening). This combination of dynamic muscle action is believed to use the stretch reflex in such a way that more than the usual number of motor units are recruited.' It should be noted, however, that the term 'plyometrics' has been casually widened by some athletes and coaches to include all jumping and bounding.

Since its introduction, two forms of plyometrics have evolved. The original version is called the shock method, in which the athlete drops down from a height and experiences a 'shock' upon landing. This, in turn, brings about a forced, involuntary eccentric contraction, which then immediately switches into a concentric contraction as the athlete jumps upwards. The landing and take-off are executed in an extremely short period of time,

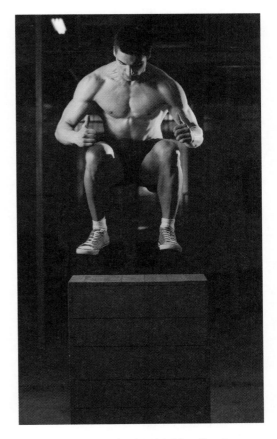

Fig. 8.2: Plyometrics is a highly effective method for athletes to improve their speed, quickness and power. (Photo: Shutterstock)

between 0.1 and 0.2sec. The shock method is the most effective method used by athletes to improve their speed, quickness and power after developing a strong strength base.

The second version of plyometrics, popular in the United States, relates to all forms of jumping, regardless of execution time. Such jumps cannot be considered truly plyometric since the intensity of execution is much lower, and the time required for making the transition from the eccentric to the concentric contraction is much greater. The term 'plyometrics' became very popular, with the publication of many books on the subject.

Plyometric Exercises

Squat jump: Squat as far as possible, and jump off the ground.

Lateral jumps: From a standing position, jump from side to side.

Power skipping: On each skip, lift the upper leg as high as possible.

Tuck jumps: With the feet shoulder-width apart, the athlete jumps, tucks their legs in, extends them, and lands.

Alternate leg bounding: Run with long strides, placing an emphasis on hang time.

Box jumps: Jump on to, and off, a large box 18in or higher.

Vertical depth jump: Starting from the top of a box, jump down and back up as fast as possible.

Plyometric push-up: Perform a normal push-up, but exert enough upward force to lift the hands and body off the ground.

Split: The split, to the contrary of what people might think, also helps plyometrics.

The concept of plyometrics was initially created by Yuri Verkhoshansky, a Soviet sports scientist who published his research in the former USSR. In 1975 Soviet athletes competing in an international competition were seen practising plyometrics as part of their warm-up, by Fred Wilt, an FBI agent and double Olympian in the 10,000m in 1948 and 1952. Wilt investigated further and discovered that Dr Michael Yessis had earlier translated Verkhoshansky's research and liaised with him to publicize the work in the West.

Since the introduction of plyometric training to the West, the risk of injury from it has been widely recognized, but it was considered that the results derived from it made it worth taking that risk. Recent research comparing plyometrics with explosive Olympic weightlifting, in terms of their training effects and consequent injuries, found that the training effects were almost identical, but that the injuries were more numerous and more serious as a consequence of plyometrics. Accordingly, on the advice of Mike Stone and Bill Sands, two recent chief physiologists at the United States Olympic Committee National Training Centre at Colorado Springs, USOC has outlawed plyometric training by athletes and coaches or at facilities under their control. Instead they recommend the use of Olympic weightlifting.

MULTIGYM

A multigym is a machine designed to provide around six to ten stations at which people may perform resistance training using fixed weights, gears or pulleys in a variety of different exercises, in order to improve their fitness. It was originally conceived in the USA in the early 1970s, by coaches wanting to assist American football players to train.

Advantages of a Multigym

Higher earning: Gym managers report considerably higher incomes from gyms that contain multigyms than from those containing free weights.

No one steals them: Multigyms are one-piece machines that weigh two tons. It is impossible to steal them without a great deal of equipment and a lot of time. Small disks in free-weight gyms are constantly stolen for a variety of purposes.

They are quiet and don't damage the floor: Casual use of free weights makes a lot of noise and can seriously damage the gym floor. Multigyms make less noise and do not damage the floor.

Easier to control: Free weights can be carried away to dark corners of the gym or even taken out of the gym. Multigyms stay put, and have a limit on the ways in which they can be used.

Easy to start using: A novice can quickly copy other users to get a good idea of the technique required for each station on a multigym. Novices using free weights need considerable coaching to lift safely.

Can help to overcome plateaus in performance: Athletes lifting weights occasionally find that their periods of progress are interrupted by 'plateaus', when that progress levels out. Using multigyms instead of free weights removes any technical or psychological issues and allows progress to resume.

Certain multigyms can be used for isokinetic (same speed) and dynamic variable resistance (same effort) training: The characteristics of multigyms are different from those of free weights, and a good coach can use these differences to the advantage of his or her athletes.

Quicker to use and change weights: An athlete who wants to vary the weight of a bar must find the spanner to remove the collar, find the weight that he or she needs, then load it on the bar and re-secure the collar on the bar. A multigym user simply moves the pin in the weight stack.

Attractive, particularly to women: Multigyms tend to be painted red, white and blue and have a lot of chrome. Whilst most men are content to use any old weights, women appreciate clean, attractive weights.

People like to use them: they encourage exercise: Whilst people associate weights with hard work, they tend to see a multigym more as a toy to play with.

They don't show up the weaker user: An athlete with a row of large disks at each end of the bar may intimidate one with an empty bar. A multigym user cannot easily see the weight being used by another user.

Requires minimal supervision: An athlete using a multigym requires little instruction or supervision. An athlete using free weights requires both instruction and supervision to ensure their safety.

Take up little space: Multigyms are difficult to move and tend to stay where they are put. Free weights tend to get spread all over the floor.

Often display helpful posters/labels: Multigyms are designed to be used in a specific way, and labels are frequently attached to them. As free weights can be used in many different ways it is not possible to display labels or posters to them.

No need for spotters: Multigym bars move up and down along a pre-determined path. The only risk of injury is putting your fingers between two weights in a stack. Free weights can fly all over the place after an accident.

Disadvantages of a Multigym

High initial cost: Multigyms can cost between £5,000 and £10,000 each. A bar with a pair of disks costs around £40.

High maintenance costs: Multigyms require regular maintenance to continue working. Nothing can be done to improve free weights, which need no such time out for maintenance.

More time out of use for maintenance: See above.

There are statistically more accidents: Research shows that there are more accidents among people using multigyms than among those using free weights.

Difficult to store: At a time where sports centres are under pressure to reinvent themselves and organize children's parties, storage is a problem. Free weights break down and can be stored in a small box.

Restricted weights available: The design of a multigym limits the minimum and maximum poundages that may be used in an exercise.

Restricted exercises available: Each multigym station is designed to be used for a specific exercise. Free weights can be used for any exercise.

Restricted movements available: The design of a multigym limits the path of every movement.

Does not help in the learning of a technique: Mimicking technique does not teach the athlete as much as specific, individual tuition.

The user may have to wait his turn to use it: Each station on a multigym is designed for just one exercise so that other athletes have to wait. Free weights can be used for any exercise.

Lack of adjustability: Only the most expensive multigyms are capable of adjustment. Free weights allow free movement.

Quickly go out of fashion: Most major chains of gym operators replace their multigyms every two or three years in order to maintain the enthusiasm of their patrons.

WEIGHTLIFTING

The lifting of heavy weights, like foot racing over short distances, is a very natural activity that every child tries at some stage of his or her development, and one that has taken place throughout the ages. There is evidence to support the fact that the sport took place in Egypt, China and Greece in ancient times, although until very recently it was considered suitable only for men aged over twenty-one years. Women, younger men and boys were considered to be at risk from lifting weights.

The formal organization and administration of the sport developed in Britain from the early 1880s, and then spread across the world; it led to the formation of the International Olympic Committee (IOC) in 1966, and the first Olympic Games in Athens, Greece. It promoted formal contests in weightlifting, the first of which took place at the Café Monico (now Boots plc) at Piccadilly Circus in Central London.

The organizers of these first formal contests had to choose from the great range of exercises that existed at that time, and they selected the fast, explosive, overhead lifts that entertained and gripped the crowds. Over time the organizers varied the exercises, then dropped weightlifting from the Games altogether until 1924, when they included the one-hand snatch, the one-hand clean and jerk, the press, the two-hands snatch and the two-hands clean and jerk.

The organizers quickly realized that the contests were lasting too long and that they were losing their audiences, so in 1928 they dropped the one-hand lifts. In 1972 they dropped the press, leaving just the snatch and the jerk. Women were included in the Olympic Games in Sydney in 2000 for the first time.

In a competition, each lifter takes three attempts in the snatch and three attempts in the jerk. The best successful attempts are then added together to produce a total, which determines the result of the competition.

Weightlifters wear simple cotton or nylon leotards. They may wear a belt and bandages on their knees, wrists and thumbs, though few choose to do so, seeing no advantage in them. The weightlifting bars used in competitions have a ring of ball-bearings that permit the ends of the bars, with the weights on them, to rotate freely and remove any strain on the wrists. The heavier weights used in competitions, those over 15kg, are made of rubber so as to avoid damage to the bar, the weights and the platform.

The International Weightlifting Federation (IWF) was established in 1905 and still exists today. It organizes all contests and maintains a register of all records.

Weightlifting is a sport that requires strength, speed, flexibility, coordination, skill and courage. It is an ideal sport for young athletes and for those working to improve their performance in other sports. Dwain Chambers used Olympic weightlifting between 1997 and 2002 when he was coached by Mike Macfarlane, before he moved over to the United States; there, his new coach converted him to powerlifting. He also started using products from the Bay Area Laboratory Company (BALCO), which resulted in him being suspended for doping in 2003. Using powerlifting and drugs, Chambers became stronger, but although he increased his muscle bulk and bodyweight, he lost some of his range of movement, which did not help him to run any faster.

No discussion on weightlifting would be complete without putting it into perspective by discussing the scale of the weights being lifted.

POWERLIFTING

In the 1950s, some weightlifters in the USA and the UK became disenchanted with the move towards the sport of Olympic weightlifting at the cost of all-round lifting. They started

WORLD RECORDS IN WEIGHTLIFTING

Men	56kg class	77kg class	105kg class
Snatch	138kg/304lb	176kg/388lb	214kg/472lb
Jerk	169kg/373lb	210kg/463lb	263kg/580lb
Women	48kg class	63kg class	75kg class
Snatch	98kg/216lb	117kg/258lb	151kg/331lb
Jerk	121kg/267lb	143kg/315lb	190kg/419lb

http://www.iwf.net/results/world-records/

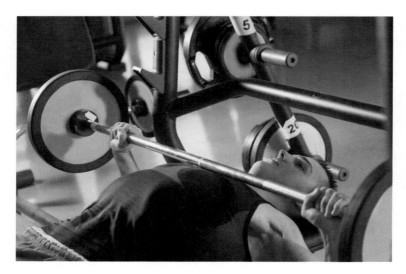

Fig. 8.3: Powerlifting is ideal for young athletes and for those working to improve their performance in other sports. (Photo: Shutterstock)

supporting a growing odd-lift movement, based on the hundreds of lifts that had grown up over the years, but which were not part of Olympic weightlifting competitions. Over the next ten years powerlifting focused on the lifts that bodybuilders used to develop the shape and outline that they required in order to prepare for a career in competitive bodybuilding in later life: the curl, the bench press and the dead lift, known as the strength set.

The curl was later dropped, as the difficulties in restricting the hip swing that permitted the use of the legs in the curl became clear. The squat was substituted for the curl. The International Powerlifting Federation (IPF) was formed in 1972. The growth of the Paralympic movement highlighted the value of the bench press for athletes unable to complete the Olympic weightlifting lifts, and it was eventually adopted for Paralympic competition in 1984.

The development of powerlifting as a sport was reflected in the battle between two large North American corporations and their presidents. Bob Hoffmann of the York Barbell Company from York, Pennsylvania, had long been using the profits of manufacturing weightlifting equipment to sponsor the sport

of weightlifting. Similarly, Ben Weider of the Weider Corporation from Montreal, Canada, had been using its profits from manufacturing weights, supplements and bodybuilding magazines to promote bodybuilding. Now both men redirected their companies to promote and sponsor powerlifting.

Powerlifting competitions comprise three attempts in the squat, bench press and dead lift, with the highest successful lift in each exercise being totalled to decide the result of the competition.

The exercises are very simple tests of extreme strength: cruel observers have described the squat as 'straightening your legs', the bench press as 'straightening your arms', and the dead lift as 'standing up straight'. It is fair, however, to state that the exercises do not promote coordination, flexibility and multi-joint movement in the same way as Olympic weightlifting.

Over the years, competitors have recognized the advantages of wearing supersuits, wide belts, specialist powerlifting boots, bandages on knees and wrists, and super-elasticated T-shirts for the bench press, and ballet shoes for the dead lift. Relying on materials such as polyester, canvas, denim, cotton and elastic to

WORLD RECORDS IN POWERLIFTING			
Men	**59kg class**	**75kg class**	**120kg= class**
Squat	295.0kg/650lb	367.5kg/810lb	485.0kg/1069lb
Bench press	200.0kg/441lb	240.0kg/529lb	370.0kg/816lb
Dead lift	275.0kg/606lb	321.0kg/708lb	397.5kg/876lb
Women	**47kg class**	**63kg class**	**84kg= class**
Squat	197.5kg/435lb	235.5kg/519lb	310.0kg/683lb
Bench press	126.0kg/278lb	166.0kg/366lb	225.5kg/497lb
Dead lift	185.5kg/409lb	245.0kg/540lb	270.5kg/596lb
http://www.powerlifting-ipf.com/44.html			

act as a brake at the end of a range of movement and to store energy has the potential for danger as it may tear and cause serious injury or even death. A few competitors have also taken prohibited drugs in order to improve performance, which can also cause serious health problems or death.

These trends have led to the organization of separate competitions for squat, bench press and dead lift, for competitors who wear supportive clothing and those who do not, and for those who use drugs and those who do not. These arrangements have also led to the establishment of around a dozen international federations to control different types of powerlifting for different types of powerlifters.

Powerlifting tends to attract athletes who have become strong participating in other sports, but who have found that they can no longer successfully compete in that sport due to losing their fitness and accumulating injuries, but that these problems do not adversely affect their success in powerlifting. Accordingly, there are fewer junior powerlifters than might be anticipated, but a far greater number of Masters' competitors than in other sports.

No discussion on powerlifting would be complete without putting it into perspective by discussing the scale of the weights being lifted.

CONCLUSION

An athlete and coach may use any method of training they wish in order to support the athlete's performance. Athletes must consider the facilities and coaches available to them, their training needs, their preferences, the cost, what best meets their needs and what they enjoy. This training will take up many hours of their lives every week for the next ten years of their lives, which makes it an important decision.

The books listed in the references at the end of this book will advise on the techniques employed in each of these training methods, and it is no part of this book to teach the sports of weightlifting and powerlifting, or the techniques of activities such as circuit training, plyometrics, weight training or speedball.

CHAPTER 9

MODERN TRAINING METHODS

by Dr Geoffrey K. Platt

In the last chapter we looked at the training methods employed by elite British sprinters over the last half century. In this chapter we will look at the scientific principles that govern all training, and against which the various training methods should be evaluated.

The components of fitness are as follows:

- strength
- speed

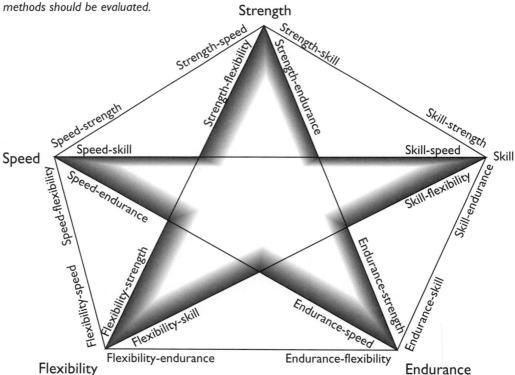

Fig. 9.1: The relationship between the components of fitness: flexibility, flexibility–endurance (Stone, Stone and Sands 2007, p.4).

- skill
- flexibility
- endurance
- body composition

The components are very closely related, and this relationship is illustrated in Fig. 9.1.

The principles of training state that in order to improve fitness, all training must meet the following criteria. It must be:

- progressive
- in overload
- varied
- planned
- specific
- reversible

GENERAL ADAPTATION TO TRAINING

The term 'general adaptation to training' was first adopted in 1956 by the Canadian biologist and endocrinologist, Hans Selye; in 1979 it was applied to resistance training and exercise conditioning by Garhammer.

After training an athlete will feel 'very sore', 'tired', 'knackered' and 'aching'. But given fluids, food and rest they will recover and even 'super-compensate', which means that they will actually improve after training. If they do not train again, this gain will be lost in a few days. Fig. 9.2 reflects this sequence.

It will be noted that these graphs have no scales on either the horizontal or vertical axes. This is because each athlete is an individual, and will recover at a different speed depending on the intensity of training and their level of fitness at the time of training.

If the athlete trains again at just the time that he or she reaches the point of super-compensation, then exactly the same process will occur, and more super-compensation will result. This can continue indefinitely, resulting in gentle but continuous progress, as shown in Fig. 9.3.

The worst case scenario is that after the first training session, as the athlete is in the trough of exhaustion, he or she trains again and gets even more tired. If this were to happen a few times, the athlete could collapse. This could mean that they twist an ankle in training due to not paying attention, or they

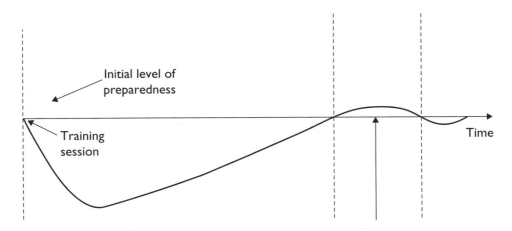

Fig. 9.2: Physiological effect of a single training session.

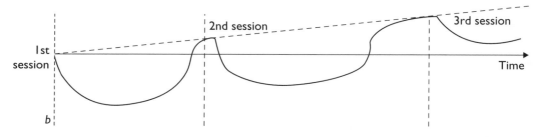

Fig. 9.3: The physiological effect of three training sessions timed to take place at the peak of super-compensation.

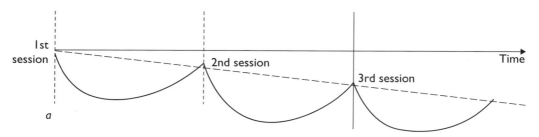

Fig. 9.4: The physiological effect of three training sessions timed to take place before recovery from the previous session.

trip over the kerb on the way home from training. This is reflected in Fig. 9.4.

By comparing the two graphs in Figs 9.3 and 9.4, it can be seen that performance may vary from gentle improvement to steady decline, or anywhere between the two, depending on the timing of subsequent training sessions.

A range of physiological and psychological tests can be performed in order to assess an athlete's recovery after training, but most coaches generally rely on feedback from the athlete. If the athlete has not recovered from the previous session by the time the next one comes round, then the coach will usually propose a gentle stretching session, rather than the athlete becoming even more exhausted and risking potential injury.

DESIGNING TRAINING PROGRAMMES

A training programme is a journey, and as in every journey, the successful traveller is the one who takes time to plan the trip and prepare for it. This is to ensure that he or she knows the starting place, the destination, and the duration of the journey, and that they have everything that is required for that journey before leaving home.

Between the end of World War II in 1945 and the fall of the Iron Curtain in 1990, the German Democratic Republic (East Germany) was the most successful sporting country that the world had ever seen. Talented athletes were identified at a very early age, sometimes as early as two or three years of age, and provided with the training and competition that they needed in order to develop.

Young athletes considered suitable for senior squads were frequently removed from competition for periods of up to a year, in order to bring them up to the fitness level of the other athletes in the squad, and for them to learn the full range of skills that they would require whilst on that squad. In this way their progression and integration into the senior squad could be completed seamlessly.

When these athletes reached puberty they were handed a computer printout setting out their daily training programme until they retired from sport, up to twenty years later. Of course, injuries and personal crises required the programme to be adjusted from time to time, but the programme was followed as closely as events permitted.

Athletes without the same resources available to them will have to adjust their aspirations, but still need to plan to the limits of those resources.

The Planning Process

SMART is a mnemonic acronym, providing criteria that act as a guide in the setting of objectives, in areas such as project management, employee performance management and personal development. It is equally valid in sporting areas. The first known use of the term occurred in the November 1981 issue of *Management Review* by George T. Doran. The principal advantage of SMART objectives is that they are easier to understand and to do, and you can then be reassured that they *have* been done.

Specific – target a specific area for improvement.
Measurable – quantify or at least suggest an indicator of progress.

Achievable – ensure that the athlete is capable of completing the work set.
Realistic – state what results can realistically be achieved, given the available resources (whilst still posing a challenge).
Time-related – specify when the result(s) can be achieved.

Clearly, all members of the coaching team need to participate in the design of these plans and targets, as they all need to have ownership of it.

The plan needs to take into consideration the following questions:

Training status: Where is the athlete now, in terms of performance? A range of fitness tests and psychological tests should be undertaken to ascertain his or her training status.

Progress: Where does the athlete need to be, in terms of performance, a) eventually and b) at the end of the training programme? The most successful athlete in the event should be assessed – and remember that by the time this athlete gets to that level of performance, standards will have increased by 10 per cent!

Exercise selection: Perform a movement analysis of the event being targeted. Consider the athlete's experience of weight training and their knowledge of technique. Check the availability of resistance-training equipment.

Training frequency and duration: Review the training frequency – the number of training sessions performed in a given time period (day or week) – and its duration – the length of time that each session lasts. Check the time that the athlete has available for strength training after all his or her other commitments.

Volume and intensity of training: Check that the volume (the amount of work performed in a given training session or time period – sets × repetitions) and the intensity (the effort with which a repetition is executed – weight lifted/personal best lift) of the proposed training is both reasonable and achievable.

Exercise order: Determine the most suitable exercise order (the sequence in which a set of repetitions is executed). The rules are:

- Power exercises, other core exercises, then assistance exercises
- Alternate 'push' and 'pull' exercises
- Finish with supersets and compound sets

Complete the session design: Do this by arranging the proposed workload into repetitions (the number of times that an exercise is undertaken) and sets (a group of repetitions undertaken without a break) and the recovery or rest interval (the time period between repetitions and sets).

Athletes today train exceptionally hard for several hours a day, but finding the time to rest and recuperate from their exertions is just as important as the actual training. It has been estimated that twice as many athletes overtrain as undertrain (Kellmann, 2002).

Sprinters go to the track in order to run there, and then go to the weights room in order to get strong. They then go home in order to continue the rehydration process that started, gently, whilst they were running, and which started in earnest as soon as they finished running. They then refuel with the food that they need.

They will then put their feet up, maybe have a nap between sessions, or just watch television or play computer games. They will go to bed and ensure that they get the eight or more hours' continuous sleep that they require after their exertions.

In short, athletes damage (in a controlled way) and break down tissue at the track or the gym, and then go home to drink, eat and rest, so as to recover from their exertions and prepare for the next session. But even this is not enough to provide the athletes with all the rest that they require in order to perform at their best in major events.

ADVANCED PROGRAMME DESIGN: PERIODIZATION

Periodization is the process by which training is broken down into blocks of weeks or months, with different objectives for each period. An example might be to divide a year into four periods, such as out of season, pre-season, start of season and competitive season.

The purpose of periodization is to adjust the quantity, quality and focus of training so as to bring the athlete to a peak of performance at the right time for an Olympic Games or a World Championships. For example, after a World Championships in August, the athlete will be ready for a rest. Four weeks' holiday, during which the athlete receives treatment for any injuries that have been troubling him or her and takes a physical and psychological break from training, leaves forty-eight weeks until the following World Championships in August the following year. If these forty-eight weeks are divided into four periods, each period could be twelve weeks (or roughly three months) long.

Between September and November, the weather is deteriorating. The athlete has taken two or three weeks' holiday and lost fitness. As the training gets more intensive year on year, the athlete will require more fitness than ever before, so the target for the out-of-competition season is to work hard to improve fitness. This will leave the athlete very tired, but as there are no races during this period, this will not be a problem.

PERIODIZATION OF A COMPETITIVE YEAR

Out of Competition	September to November	Fitness and training
Pre-season	December to February	Strength build-up
Start of season	March to May	Power build-up
Competitive season	June to August	Power maintenance

Between December and February the weather is often very poor. The athlete is now fit and ready to go. The strength build-up training is very exhausting and may leave him very weak in the short term, but this is not a problem as there are no races at this time of year.

From March to May the weather is starting to improve. The athlete now focuses on power build-up, when power is strength and speed. As the athlete has already been working on strength for ten weeks, the focus is on improving speed. The athlete will be doing less work, be less tired and getting faster. This will be useful as the season is now starting, with club and county championships.

Between June and August the summer has arrived. The athlete is now maintaining the power that he or she has already achieved. The work should not be troubling him, and he should be ready to race. As the period progresses, performances will improve so that the athlete is at a peak at the end of the period at the World Championships.

Of course, track work will continue throughout the year, but the volume and intensity is such that it will not substantially affect the fitness and performance of the athlete.

The names of the periods are only a guide, and the fact that these names do not completely reflect what is happening on the track does not matter. The seasons reflect what is generally happening on the track, and setting the periods against the calendar is an arbitrary judgement.

A training cycle of the type that has been discussed in this chapter is generally called a macrocycle, and lasts somewhere between a few months and the four years of an Olympic cycle. A macrocycle may be divided into two or more mesocycles. In the case of an Olympic athlete, the macrocycle can be the four-year Olympic cycle, and the meso-cycles will probably be the individual years of the cycle. These mesocycles may be divided into two or more microcycles, each lasting between one and four weeks.

As can be seen, periodization is a very complex subject and many models exist for different situations and different athletes. Considerable volumes have been written on the subject, but this chapter merely introduces the subject to athletes and coaches, rather than covering it in detail.

WARMING UP

All training must be preceded by a warm-up so as to reduce the risk of injury and to prepare the athlete for maximal exercise.

A warm-up is a programme of exercises designed to assist the body to adjust from a state of rest (or comparative rest) to a state of increased exertion. It is usually performed at the start of an exercise session, but may also be performed at any other time before the exertion ends, where there is an increase in intensity.

An example of where a warm-up may be

required mid-session would be where an athlete undertook a technique session whilst fresh and alert, and then wanted to fit in a high intensity session at the end in order to work on incorporating the newly learnt techniques into a realistic competitive practice. The technique work may not have prepared the athlete for the high intensity session, so a further warm-up is necessary in order to avoid the risk of injury.

The objectives of a warm-up are:

- to raise the body temperature
- to stretch the muscles, so as to move the heat around the body
- to prepare for exercise mentally

The reasons for warming up are:

- to prepare the mind and body for activity
- to prevent injury
- to improve performance

A warm-up should prepare the following systems for exertion:

- the brain
- the cardiovascular system, of heart, lungs and blood vessels
- the muscular system

Because a warm-up is usually at the start of the day or the start of a session, it may also be a social event which brings athletes and coaches together and arouses all concerned, so as to motivate them to higher levels of performance. This may be in the form of a short game of football or basketball, or simply as a group activity led by a coach.

The duration of a warm-up depends on:

- the intensity of the planned session
- the duration of the planned session
- the condition of the participants before the session

- the environmental conditions, such as temperature and humidity

It should generally last between ten and thirty minutes.

Pulse-Raising Activities

If your athletes have had a night partying and are suffering the effects of over-indulgence, then you should start very slowly and carefully with some of the following exercises:

- walking
- heel-toe walking
- pitter patter
- striding
- jogging
- skipping
- side stepping facing the right
- side stepping facing the left
- stretched out side stepping facing the right
- stretched out side stepping facing the left
- jogging with the knees up
- jogging whilst kicking your bum
- repeat everything facing backwards
- two feet together, bunny hopping
- knees up to the waist bounding
- touch the ground, then bound
- sprints
- sprints from a lying start

Stretching

Stretching should not, under any circumstances, be confused with mobility training. Stretching is about achieving results less than, but close to, your best; mobilizing is about improving your range of movement in order to achieve better results than you have ever done before. Stretching will rely on exercises with which the athlete is familiar; mobility training will frequently introduce new exercises.

If the stretching session is under the supervision of a professional strength and conditioning coach, then it will be carefully structured and planned; otherwise it is frequently arranged so as to work from the head to the toes, so as to avoid missing out any part of the body. An understanding of the anatomy of the bones, joints and muscles is very useful when planning a stretching programme.

Mental Preparation

It is useful if the athlete knows the exact time the session will start and the programme that it will follow, so that he or she can give some thought to it, the problems that it will cause them, what will go well and what may not go so well. A professional athlete may well have a professional sports psychologist who will prepare a script to get them aroused and motivated for the session ahead.

WARMING DOWN

There are two particular problems that need to be dealt with during warming down. The first is that some athletes find it useful to become aggressive in order to perform at their best, but aggressive behaviour can cause problems if the athlete uses inappropriate language or uses or threatens violence; therefore particular attention needs to be made to calm them in the warming-down session.

The second problem is that load-bearing and compressive activity, such as lifting weights, bounding or sprinting, can compress the spine, so the athlete can lose up to 2in in height during a session.

The objectives of a warm-down are:

■ to lower the body temperature
■ to stretch the muscles and joints
■ to mentally calm the athlete after exercise

The reasons for warming down are:

■ to prepare the mind and body to stop activity
■ to prevent muscle stiffness and soreness
■ to return the body to its resting state

A warm-down should prepare the following systems for relaxing rest:

■ the brain
■ the cardiovascular system, of heart, lungs and blood vessels
■ the muscular system

SPRINT DRILLS

Sprint drills improve the sprinter's skills and reduce weaknesses that may cause injury.

There is no doubt that time spent on warming up and cooling down will improve an athlete's level of performance and accelerate the recovery process needed before training or competing again. An element of the warm-up programme should include event-specific drills to stimulate the appropriate neuromuscular action for the range of movement and correct posture.

Drills should be conducted wearing trainers and not spikes. In all the drills, the coach/athlete should ensure a tall and relaxed posture with a correct range of movement of the arms. Check for the following:

■ Eyes focused at the end of the lane – tunnel vision
■ Head in line with the spine – held high and square
■ Face relaxed – jelly jaw – no tension – mouth relaxed
■ Chin down, not out
■ Shoulders down (long neck), relaxed and square in the lane at all times

- Back straight (not hunched)
- Abdominals braced (not tummy pulled in)
- Smooth forward/backward action of the arms, not across the body – drive back with elbows – brush vest with elbows – hands move from shoulder height to hips for men and from bust height to hips for ladies
- Elbows held at 90 degrees at all times (angle between upper arm and lower arm)
- Hands relaxed, fingers loosely curled, thumb uppermost
- Hips remain stable during the execution of the drills

General Sprint Drills

The following exercises are examples of general sprint drills.

HIGH KNEES

Aims: To improve overall coordination, increase hip range of motion, challenge the hip flexors, and improve ground contact explosiveness.
Amount: Two repetitions over 20 to 30m.
Action: Travel forwards by slightly leaning forwards, pumping the arms and driving the knees high with dorsi-flexed toes (flexed upward) in front of the body. Be sure to drive the hands/arms to counterbalance the body, and only contact the ground with the ball of the foot.

STRAIGHT LEGS

Aim: To develop the muscles of the backside and the hamstrings.
Amount: Two repetitions over 20 to 30m.
Action: Lock the legs straight and point the toes. Step out down the track.

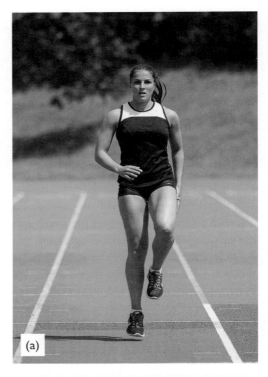
(a)

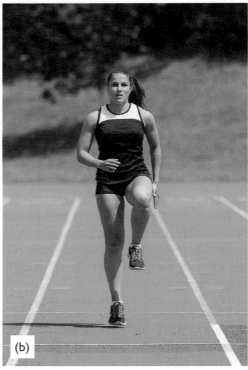
(b)

Fig. 9.5 (a-f): Sequence showing high knees drills. (Photos: Darren Charles Holloway)

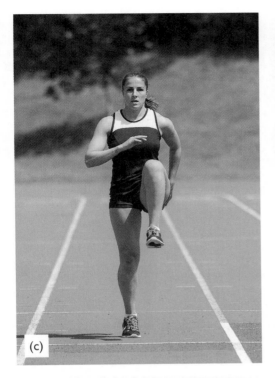

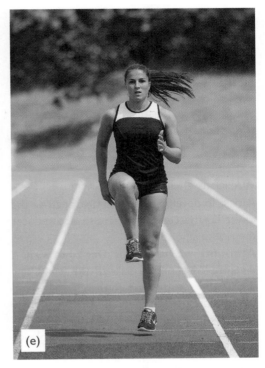

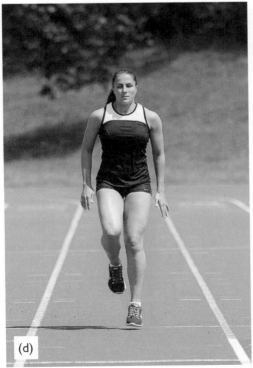

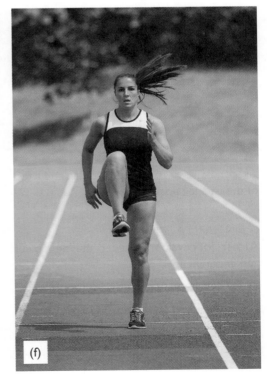

HEEL KICKS/BUTT KICKS

Aim: To develop correct leg sprint action in the mid-section following the drive off the rear leg.

Amount: Two repetitions over 20 to 30m.

Action: Fast leg movement on the balls of the feet – drive the knee up and bring the heel to the underside of the backside and the thigh parallel with the ground.

WALKING ON TOES

Aims: To develop balance and strengthen the lower leg muscles (this exercise also reduces the risk of shin splints).

Amount: Two repetitions over 20 to 30m.

Action: Walk on the balls of the feet, lifting the free leg so that the thigh is parallel with the ground, the lower leg is vertical and the toes dorsi-flexed (this end position can be held for a second or two to develop balance and a feel of the free leg position).

WALKING ON HEELS

Aims: To develop balance and strengthen the lower leg muscles (this exercise also reduces the risk of shin splints).

Amount: Two repetitions over 20 to 30m.

Action: Walk on the heels of the feet, lifting free leg so that the thigh is parallel with the ground, the lower leg is vertical and the toes dorsi-flexed (this end position can be held for a second or two to develop balance and a feel of the free leg position).

SPRINT ARM ACTION

Aims: To develop shoulder muscle power and endurance.

Amount: 10 to 20sec.

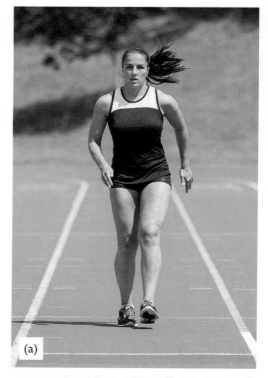
(a)

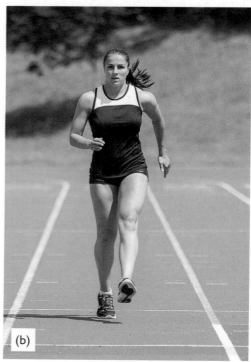
(b)

Fig. 9.6 (a-f): Sequence showing straight leg drills. (Photos: Darren Charles Holloway)

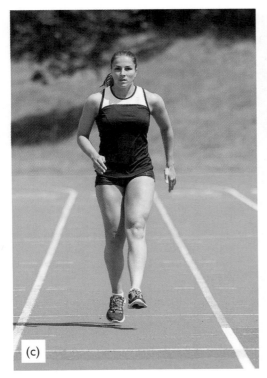

(c)

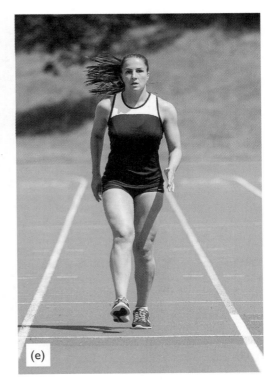

(e)

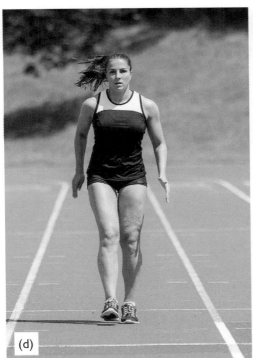

(d)

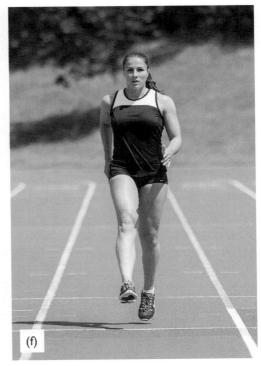

(f)

Fig. 9.7 (a-j): Sequence showing heel kicks drills. (Photos: Darren Charles Holloway)

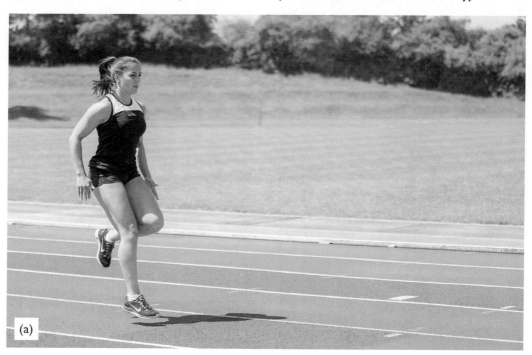

(a)

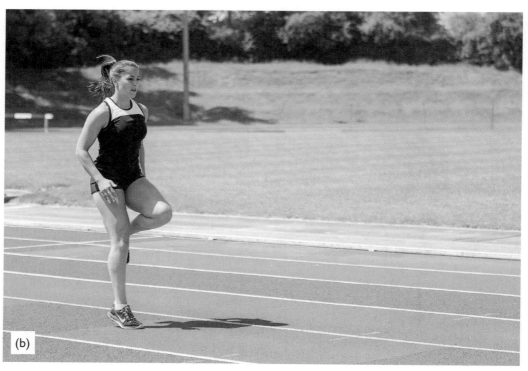

(b)

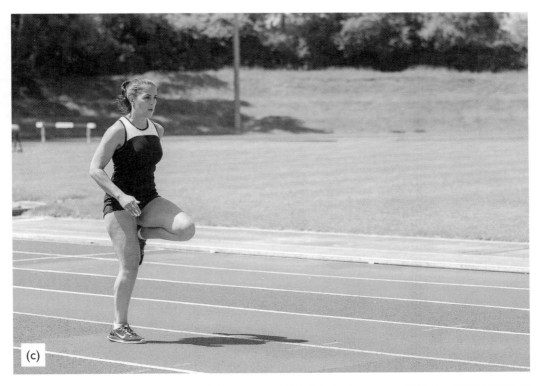

(c)

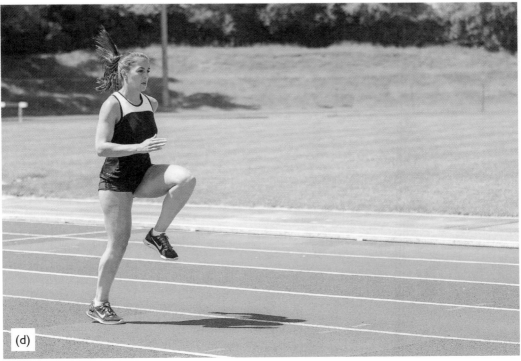

(d)

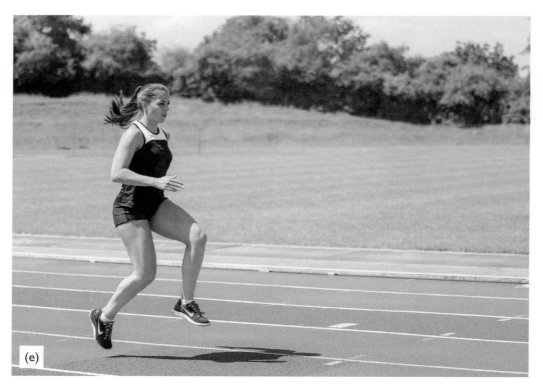

(e)

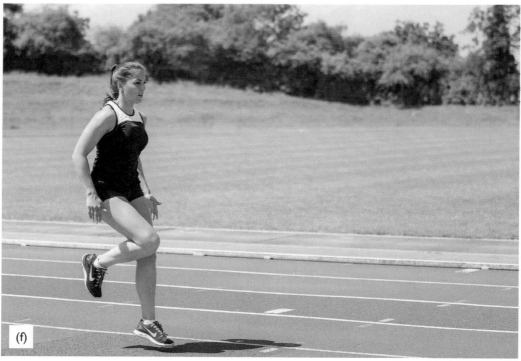

(f)

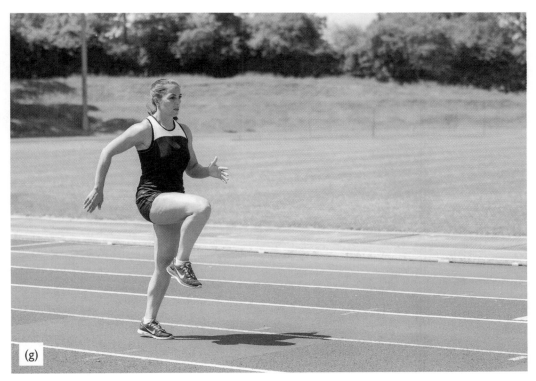

(g)

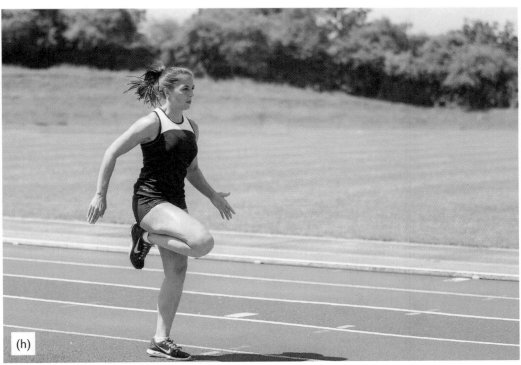

(h)

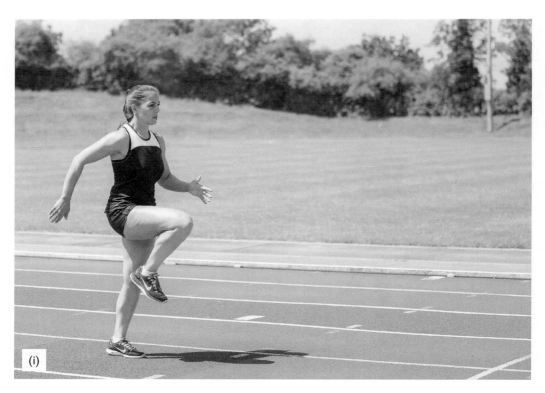

(i)

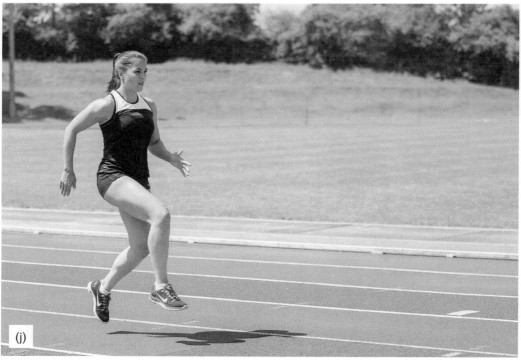

(j)

Action: Assume the lunge position, brace the abdominals, maintain a straight back, use a fast sprint arm action.

LEG CYCLING

Aims: To develop the correct leg sprint action and strengthen the hamstring muscles.
Amount: 10 to 20sec on each leg.
Action: Stand next to a wall or rail that you can hold on to so as to maintain balance, stand tall, brace the abdominals; stand on the leg nearest the wall, lift the thigh of the other leg so it is parallel with the ground, the lower leg vertical and toes dorsi-flexed, sweep the leg down and under your body, pull the heel up into the buttocks, cycle the leg through to the front, pull the toes up, bring the upper thigh through to be parallel with the ground, and extend the lower leg; then commence the next cycle.

LEG DRIVES

Aims: To develop hip flexor strength and speed.
Amount: 10 to 20sec for each leg.
Action: Stand facing a wall with your hands on the wall at chest height, position your feet so that the body is straight and at 45 degrees to the wall, keep your neck in line with your spine (head up), bring one leg up so the thigh is parallel with the ground, with the lower leg vertical and the toes dorsi-flexed (the starting position), then drive the foot down towards the ground, and as the toes make contact with the ground, quickly pull the foot up and return the leg to its starting position.

SKIPS

Aim: To develop correct leg and foot action in preparation for the foot strike.
Amount: Two repetitions over 20 to 30m.
Action: Skip on the balls of the feet, lifting the free leg so that the thigh is parallel with the ground, the lower leg is vertical and the toes dorsi-flexed.

SIDE STRIDES CROSSOVER

Aims: To increase flexibility and the range of hip movement.
Amount: Two repetitions over 20 to 30m.
Action: A steady jog sideways on the balls of the feet – right leg across the front of the left leg, left leg across the back of the right leg, right leg across the back of the left leg, left leg across the front of right leg; then repeat this sequence.

SKIP AND CLAP

Aims: To increase flexibility and the range of horizontal leg movement.
Amount: Two repetitions over 20 to 30m.
Action: Skip on the balls of the feet – bring the whole leg up so it is horizontal with the ground with the toes dorsi-flexed, and at the same time clap the hands together under the leg. The arms then come back up to the side to form a crucifix.

SKIP CLAW

Aim: To develop the drive-down action of the leading leg.
Amount: Two repetitions over 20 to 30m.
Action: Skip on the balls of the feet – bring the leg up so the thigh is at least horizontal with the ground, with the lower leg vertical and the toes dorsi-flexed, then drive the foot down so that the ball of the foot strikes the ground below the hip.

SKIP FOR HEIGHT

Aim: To develop rear leg drive.
Amount: Two repetitions over 20 to 30m.
Action: Skip on the balls of the feet – the emphasis is on the rear leg drive and driving back the elbow; lift the free leg so that the thigh is parallel with the ground, the lower leg is vertical and the toes dorsi-flexed.

CHEST PASS

Aims: To develop shoulder and chest strength and speed.

Amount: 10 to 20sec.

Action: Stand approximately 2m away from and facing a wall, holding a light medicine ball (2–5kg) in your hands on its sides: with the knees relaxed, the abdominals braced and keeping the back straight, push the ball powerfully away against the wall, and meet the rebound with bent arms and hands ready to push the ball back immediately (do not catch then push back).

SPEED HOPS

Aim: To develop the reactive ability of the leg muscles.

Amount: 10 to 20sec on each leg.

Action: With the abdominals braced, keeping the back straight and looking forwards (not down), hop on the spot keeping the legs relatively straight (the knees should not be locked): as the ball of the foot lands, push explosively back up – minimize knee bend on landing.

SPEED HOPS LEG CYCLING

Aim: To develop fast sprint leg-cycling action – see the Leg Cycling exercise above.

Amount: Five hops on each leg.

Action: Brace the abdominals, keep the back straight and look forwards (not down): hop forwards on one leg, pulling the heel up into the buttocks; cycle the leg through to the front, pulling the toes up; bring the upper thigh through to be parallel with the ground, then extend the lower leg and land on the ball of the foot; immediately explode back up and commence the next cycle.

RUN-OUTS

Aim: To develop a tall, relaxed and smooth sprint action.

Amount: Six repetitions over 40m.

Action: Tip start and gradual build-up of speed over the 40m: the first two reps focus on a tall action, the next two on tall and relaxed, and the last two on tall, relaxed and smooth.

CHAPTER 10

FITNESS TESTING FOR SPRINTING

by Dr Geoffrey K. Platt

A fitness test is a test conducted to assess an athlete's performance against one of the components of physical fitness. An objective test of fitness usually requires testing each component independently under standardized laboratory conditions, although field-based testing may also prove useful. A test should only be conducted with the approval of the subject, who should be fully informed of the reasons for performing it, and the primary consideration during the test should be their safety. It is important that the tester ensures that he or she knows of any illness, injury, medication or treatment affecting the subject at the time of the test, so that the risk to health is minimized. Equipment and test procedures must be safe.

The components of fitness are:

- strength
- speed
- power
- flexibility
- endurance
- body composition

The components are very closely related, and this relationship is illustrated in the diagram (see Fig. 10.1).

In the same way that a coach seeks an objective assessment of their athlete's technique through performance analysis, and an assessment of their mental condition by a sports psychiatrist, so they want an objective assessment of their physical fitness by regular fitness testing, preferably conducted by an independent sports scientist under standardized laboratory conditions.

Armed with objective and up-to-date assessments of the athlete's physical fitness, technique and mental condition, a coach can make accurate and effective decisions, both in training and in competition, which will result in medals and records.

As in all coaching matters, the primary objective must be the safety and protection of the athlete. With this in mind, the athlete should be told the reasons for the testing, the tests should be explained, and his or her consent sought for the testing to take place. The tester should then make all reasonable enquiries into the health and fitness of the athlete, including details of all illnesses, injuries, medications and treatments, and then take all necessary precautions to ensure their safety. A PAR-Q is the name given to a participation questionnaire designed specifically to determine the fitness of a sports participant: it is a useful tool in this process, and both British and American versions are given below.

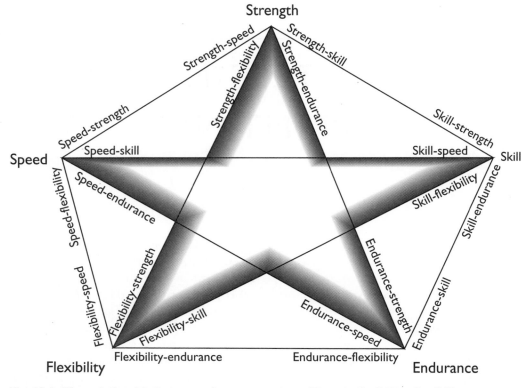

Fig. 10.1: The relationship between the components of fitness; flexibility, flexibility–endurance (Stone, Stone and Sands 2007, p.4).

STRENGTH

The definition of strength is the ability of a muscle or system of muscles to lift a maximum weight, overcome a maximum resistance, or exert a maximum force. Strength is essential for movement to take place. The amount of strength generated in a muscle or group of muscles depends on the type of action, the speed of the movement, and the length of the muscle or muscles. Although initial gains in strength are largely determined by neural factors, such as muscle activation, longer term gains usually rely on increases in muscle size, called hypertrophy.

Strength is frequently assessed in terms of absolute strength, dynamic strength, elastic strength, explosive strength, relative strength, specific strength, starting strength, strength deficit, strength endurance and static strength, and one repetition maximum (1RM – the highest weight that an athlete can lift once).

The term 'strength' relates to physical strength, not to mental strength or strength of will, as some students suspect.

Examples of sportsmen who require strength include weightlifters and wrestlers; examples of athletes who require strength include shot putters and hammer throwers.

Participants in track and field athletics, even those in the throwing events, do not require great strength. However, they do need to undertake strength training in order to

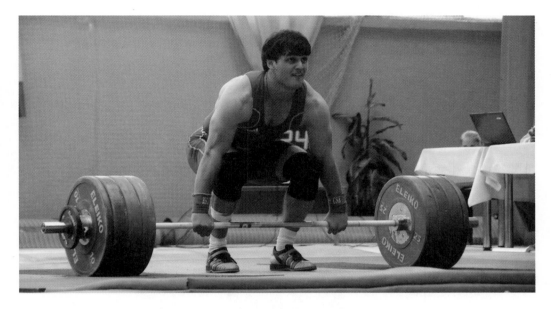

Fig. 10.2: Weightlifters require strength. (Photo: Shutterstock)

eliminate weaknesses or muscle imbalances that may cause injuries and restrict their participation in competition or training, and therefore affect their ability to win medals at major championships.

Those who compete in the jumps or on the track require good strength-to-(body)weight ratios and therefore need to refrain from adding bulk, even muscle bulk that will diminish their ability to run quickly or jump good distances. British sprinters such as Dwain Chambers and Harry Aikinees-Areetey, who are naturally strong and possess exceptional natural physiques, have had to take advice from some of the best strength and conditioning specialists in the country in order to avoid gaining additional muscle and therefore bodyweight.

Strength Testing

Strength takes months to develop, so it is sufficient to test an athlete's strength every

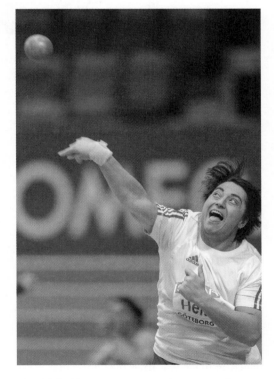

Fig. 10.3: Shot putters require strength. (Photo: Shutterstock)

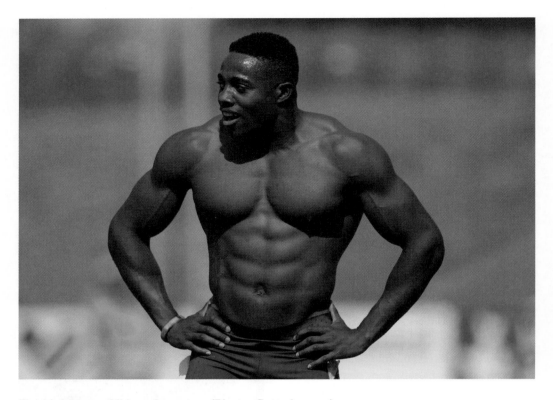

Fig. 10.4: Harry Aikines-Aryeetey. (Photo: Getty Images)

six months unless he or she has suffered a serious injury and there is a need to assess his or her rehabilitation more regularly.

Testing should be carried out by a sports scientist, a strength and conditioning coach or a personal coach, who has a working knowledge of anatomy and who is familiar with the tests and the equipment. The testing should not be rushed.

To be a true strength test, the athlete should be tested on their one repetition maximum (1RM).

There are a vast number of muscles in the human body and a coach or scientist wanting to obtain meaningful results needs to carefully consider which muscles to test, according to which muscles will have the most impact on athletic performance, and which muscles have been the focus of recent training.

The choice of equipment will be largely governed by the equipment available. Universities will have cybex isokinetic machines, capable of measuring hip and leg strength, but these cost approximately £25,000 each, so few other places will have them. A leg and back dynamometer performs a very similar test and will get an almost identical result, at a cost of only £337.00 plus VAT, but there are no more of them available (these prices are current at the time of writing).

A complete and accurate record should be kept of all testing, and the results obtained, and it should be stored in a safe place where it can be easily accessed in subsequent years.

The ways to improve strength are discussed in Chapter 9, Modern Training Methods.

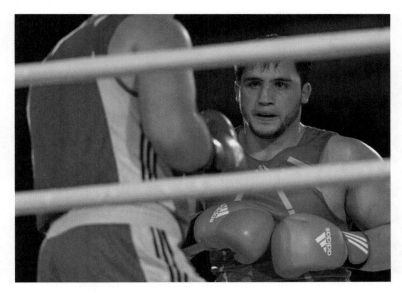

Fig. 10.5: Boxers need speed of movement. (Photo: Shutterstock)

SPEED

Speed may be defined as the distance travelled in a given time; in sport this is usually measured in metres per second (it is a scalar quantity). In walking, running and sprinting, speed is a product of stride length and stride rate (stride length × stride rate). Speed is also the ability to perform a movement quickly. Speed of movement of either the whole body (as in sprinting) or of part of the body is frequently an important component of sports performance.

Examples of sportsmen who require speed include boxers and baseball players; examples of athletes who require speed include javelin throwers and relay runners.

Speed is the result of all the other components of fitness. When an athlete possesses the flexibility to increase his or her stride length, the strength to accelerate sharply, the endurance to complete the distance, and a good body composition, then speed will result.

Start Speed

The time that it takes a sprinter to react to the gun and get to maximum speed can be broken down into several segments:

- Thinking time (deciding what to do)
- Reaction time (reacting to the gun and starting to move)
- Acceleration time (powering into one's stride and up to top speed)

Most sprinters will have given some thought as to the way in which they will react when they hear the gun. It has been said that sprinters should go on the 'B' of the 'Bang'. Most sprinters will brace both legs against the starting blocks and drive themselves down the track. If the athlete has prepared properly, then thinking time will occur before the gun goes and the clock starts.

Nowadays the gun is not a regular firearm, but a machine that sends the sound of a gunshot to a speaker in each of the starting blocks used by the athletes. This means that every athlete hears the sound at exactly the

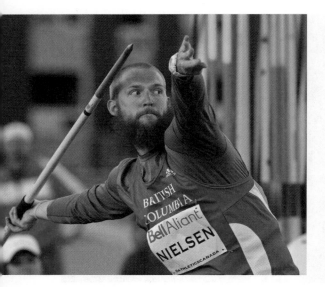

Fig. 10.6: Javelin thrower. (Photo: Shutterstock)

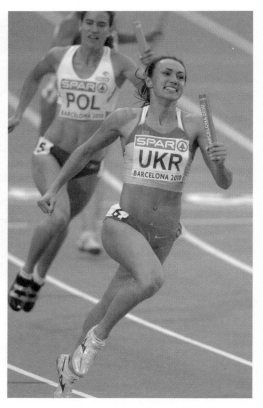

Fig. 10.7: Relay runners. (Photo: Shutterstock)

same time and therefore avoids any of them securing an advantage by being a little closer to the starter. IAAF rules stipulate that the 'gun' also receives a signal back from the starting blocks as soon as the sprinter braces against them.

If the athlete reacts in under 0.1sec then he or she is deemed to have anticipated the gun and is adjudged to have made a false start (most athletes actually react around 0.13sec after the gun). The first time in a race that an athlete makes a false start, then all the athletes in the race are warned; the second time that an athlete false starts in the same race, then he or she is disqualified. Modern electronic timers are capable of measuring all events to the nearest one millionth of a second.

A coach may use a competition 'gun' and starting blocks to measure the reaction time of an athlete. Two or three decimal places may be used in order to increase the accuracy of the testing. Each athlete should be permitted three attempts in order to eliminate the risk of their making a technical error in starting.

There are three other ways of measuring the athlete's reaction time:

- Timing gates used in the study of sports science at universities can measure the time taken to move from point A (the blocks) to point B (at 1m) (see Fig. 10.17). They have the advantage that they can also measure the speed of acceleration or at any other stage of a race.
- Reaction time is used in psychology and sports science. Lights are illuminated in a random order and the subject reacts by pressing a button of the same colour as the light.

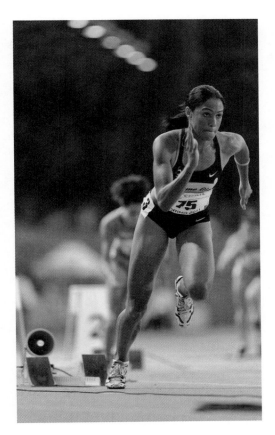

Fig. 10.8: Electronic starting blocks. (Photo: Shutterstock)

■ Ruler drop, where the athlete sits on a chair positioned next to a table, with his forearm resting on the table. A ruler or rod is suspended next to his or her extended hand and the athlete is instructed to catch the ruler as soon as he notices that it has been released. The distance which the ruler has dropped before it is caught is a measure of the reaction time of the athlete.

Acceleration time can be measured between any two distances chosen by the coach, such as from 5m to 30m. These distances will usually be determined by the age, height, strength and gender of the athlete. Timing gates can be used to measure the time taken, or, if these are not available, then a simple stop watch, as used by every coach, provides a useful alternative (see Fig. 10.9).

POWER

Power is the product of strength and speed (power = strength × speed) and therefore a combination of two components of fitness, rather than a component of fitness in its own right. Scientists define power as the rate at which energy is expended or work is done, and measure it in watts (W) (power = work done/time taken). Power is the decisive component for most athletic activities. A powerful athlete has to be able to transform physical energy into force at a fast rate. This ability depends on the amount of ATP produced per unit time. Sprinting, jumping and throwing events are activities requiring great power and very high rates of ATP production.

Examples of sportsmen who require strength include weightlifters and shot putters. As power = strength × speed, both of these are power athletes. The weightlifter is lifting an extremely heavy weight as quickly as he can, but because it is a very heavy weight, he is not moving very quickly in absolute terms. The shot putter is throwing a much lighter object a great deal faster.

The Sargent Jump

The sargent jump is the best test for power. To undertake this test requires a wall, a tape measure, a stepladder, chalk and an assistant, though it can be conducted with just a wall and a piece of chalk; so it is also the cheapest and easiest test.

The test is conducted as follows:

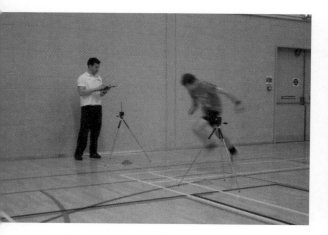

Fig. 10.9: Timing gates.

- The athlete warms up for 10min
- The athlete chalks the end of his/her finger tips
- The athlete stands side on to the wall; keeping both feet on the ground, he/she reaches up as high as possible with one hand and marks the wall with the tips of the fingers (M1)
- The athlete from a static position jumps as high as possible and marks the wall with the chalk on his fingers (M2)
- The assistant measures and records the distance between M1 and M2
- The athlete repeats the test three times
- The assistant calculates the average of the recorded distances and uses this value to assess the athlete's performance

FLEXIBILITY

Flexibility is the capacity to perform joint actions through a wide range of movement. Examples of sportsmen who require mobility include gymnasts and dancers; athletes who require endurance include hurdlers and high jumpers.

The advantages of flexibility training are

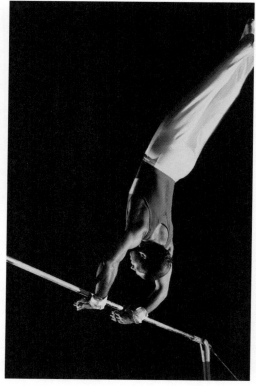

Fig. 10.10: Gymnasts need to be flexible. (Photo: Shutterstock)

that it prevents injury, maximizes potential and assists in the learning technique. The athlete should train for flexibility at the start of training, and at the start of a session.

Flexibility is achieved through static stretching – active and passive – and ballistic stretching.

Static Stretching

Active: The person stretching supplies the force for the stretch. The end position is held for different lengths of time (usually about 30sec). It is easy to learn and effective, it does not elicit the stretch reflex, and there is less chance of injury.

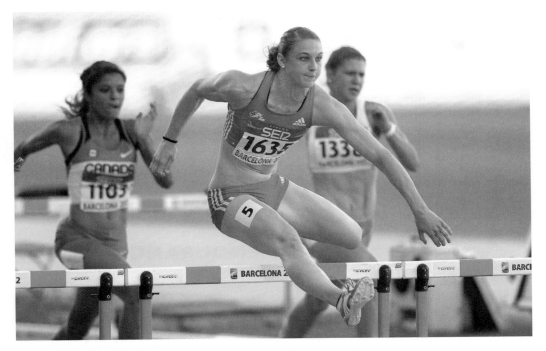

Fig. 10.11: Hurdlers also need flexibility. (Photo: Shutterstock)

Passive: A partner or device is used to provide the force for the stretch. It is usually possible to achieve a greater degree of stretch with passive stretching than with active stretching.

PNF (Proprioceptive Neuromuscular Facilitation): This stretch uses an experienced partner to passively stretch the muscle, and combines alternating contraction and relaxation of both agonist and antagonist muscles. The effect is to cause neural responses (that inhibit the contraction of the muscle being stretched) to be switched off. PNF positively affects the strength of the muscle.

Ballistic Stretching

This involves a bouncing movement in which the end position is not held. In ballistic stretching, the momentum of the moving limb may cause the joint to be forced beyond its normal and safe range of motion. A dynamic movement is used to create ballistic movement in order to stretch the agonist, but this results in initiation of the stretch reflex by the muscle spindles causing the stretched muscle to contract, thereby providing resistance to the stretch. It is usually only performed on the lower body and after a comprehensive warm-up involving static and dynamic flexibility.

There are thirteen factors that influence flexibility:

- Age (and stage of development)
- Gender (women are more flexible than men!)
- Joint laxity (the extensibility of ligaments supporting the joint)
- Muscle balance and the strength of the muscles

- Muscle hypertrophy, or any skin or tissue folds such as a 'spare tyre'
- Structural barriers of joint construction and bones
- The ability of the neuromuscular system to inhibit or create contraction in the antagonist muscles, for example reciprocal inhibition, stretch reflex, inverse stretch reflex
- The athlete's internal and external environment
- Recent injury to the muscle or joint
- Inappropriate or tight clothing
- Adaptation to habitual posture
- Some movements require a high degree of skill
- The elasticity and extensibility of the muscles, tendons and connective tissues of those muscles being stretched

The Rules of Stretching

- Do not force a stretch to the point of pain
- Never stretch when taking medication for pain
- Flexibility must be developed slowly, particularly after injury
- Older people should take more care when stretching
- Avoid vigorous stretching following a long period of immobilization (sling or cast)
- Avoid stretching swollen joints and over-stretching weak muscles
- Exercise great care when applying a passive stretch to a partner (be slow and ask for feedback)
- PNF techniques are not always suitable for people with high blood pressure (isometric contractions may increase arterial blood pressure excessively)
- Beginners should use static stretching techniques

- Well trained athletes who use ballistic stretching should precede this type of stretching with static stretching

There is a whole range of flexibility exercises that cover all areas of the body, and which may all be used as tests of flexibility. This chapter is not large enough to adequately describe a worthwhile number of these, so readers are referred to *The Science of Flexibility* by Michael J. Alter (published by Human Kinetics Publishing).

ENDURANCE

Endurance is the ability to sustain an activity for a prolonged period of time. Endurance has two main components: cardiorespiratory endurance, which is particularly important in whole body activities, and muscular endurance, which is particularly important in activities involving individual muscles. Sports scientists investigating functional systems have found it useful to divide endurance into short-term endurance (35sec to 2min), medium-term endurance (2–10min), and long-term endurance (over 10min). Success in endurance activities is generally associated with high VO2 max, a high lactate threshold, high economy of effort, and a high percentage of slow-twitch fibres.

Examples of sportsmen who require endurance include triathletes and long-distance swimmers; athletes who require endurance include marathon runners and long-distance track runners.

Expired Air Analysis

An athlete's endurance and the efficiency of his or her cardiovascular respiration can be assessed in a range of ways. Expired air

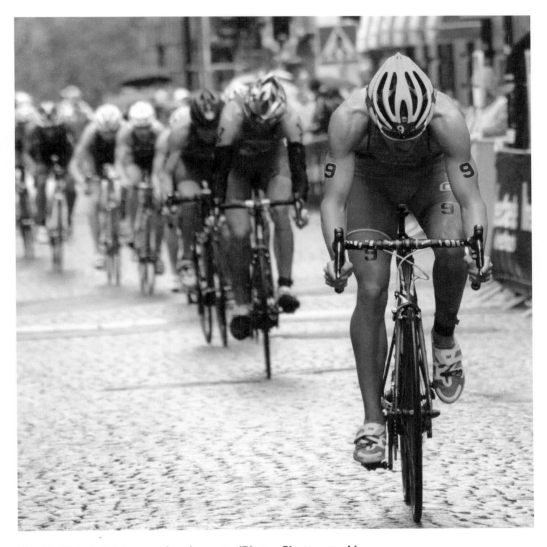

Fig. 10.12: Triathletes need endurance. (Photo: Shutterstock)

analysis (both computerized and manual looks at the percentage of oxygen used and the amount of carbon dioxide exhaled.

Blood lactate tests can determine the lactate threshold, and blood-pressure monitors (Fig. 10.14) can assist in identifying stress during training.

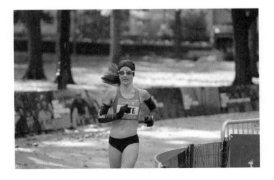

Fig. 10.13: Endurance is essential for a marathon runner. (Photo: Shutterstock)

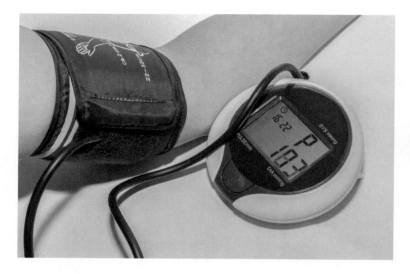

Fig. 10.14: Blood-pressure monitor. (Photo: Shutterstock)

Heart-rate monitors are useful in assisting coaches and athletes to remain in the 70 to 90 per cent of maximum training load needed to maintain the training effect. Stopwatches are useful when conducting physiological testing as well as during training.

BODY COMPOSITION

Body composition may be defined as the components of the human body described as a percentage of the total body mass. Essentially sports scientists divide bodyweight into lean bodyweight and fat mass. Examples of sportsmen who require mobility include shot putters and endurance runners.

There are four methods of measuring body composition. The most accurate method is the body pod (Fig. 10.15), where the athlete needs to undress and submerse themselves in water in order to measure his or her volume and bodyweight and therefore calculate body composition.

The next most accurate method is the quickest and easiest test, using bodyfat calipers. The calipers 'pinch an inch' of bodyfat from the the bicep, the tricep, supra-iliac

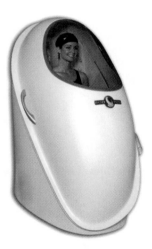

Fig. 10.15: A body pod.

(above the hip) and sub-scapula (under the shoulder blade). The four results are then input into tables or computers to calculate the overall body composition.

The third method is electrical impedence, where the athlete holds the meter between the two hands, so that an electrical current passes around the body so that body composition may be measured and quickly displayed on the screen. Some people feel a slight electric shock when undertaking this test.

The final method is body mass index, the least accurate method and, ironically, the one used by doctors when calculating body composition. The athlete is measured and weighed, and the results inserted in the following formula:

$$BMI = \frac{Bodyweight\ in\ kg}{Height\ in\ metres^2}$$

PERSONAL FITNESS PROFILE

Personal Fitness Profile	
Name	
Address	
Postcode	
Telephone number	
Height	Bodyfat biceps
Chest	Bodyfat triceps
Hips	Bodyfat sub-scapula
Weight	Bodyfat supra-iliac
Waist	Bodyfat %

Nutrition
(One sentence to describe each meal in general terms, and one sentence on how you compare with the rest of the class and how you feel that you can improve.)

Strength
(One sentence to describe the test carried out. One sentence on the result. One sentence on how you compare with the rest of the class.)

Endurance
(One sentence to describe the test carried out. One sentence on the result. One sentence on how you compare with the rest of the class.)

Fitness
(One sentence to describe the test carried out. One sentence on the result. One sentence on how you compare with the rest of the class.)

Speed
(One sentence to describe the test carried out. One sentence on the result. One sentence on how you compare with the rest of the class.)

Flexibility
(One sentence to describe the test carried out. One sentence on the result. One sentence on how you compare with the rest of the class.)

Name **Age** **Date**

Resting heart rate (for 10sec and 60sec)	
Maximal heart rate (220 - age in years)	
Working heart rate (mhr - rhr)	
Minimum heart rate (whr × 60%) = rhr	
Upper limit heart rate (whr × 80%) = rh.r	

During exercise **After exercise**

1		1	
2		2	
3		3	
4		4	
5		5	
6		6	
7		7	
8		8	
9		9	
10		10	
11			
12			
13			
14			
15			
16			
17			
18			
19			
20			

My Plan

(Select one or two or the above areas that particularly need improvement and propose the ways in which you intend to go about it).

Signed _____   Date _____

Fitness Questionnaire (UK)

All questions must be answered. Your answers will be used as the basis for our advice. Please supply the name and address as you want it to appear on your certificate.

Name

Address

Age   **Occupation**

Sports that you participate in

Sports that you coach

	Yes	No
1. Do you have heart disease, high blood pressure or any other cardio-vascular problems?		
2. Is there a history of heart disease in your family?		
3. Do you ever have pains in your heart and chest, especially associated with minimal effort?		
4. Do you often get headaches, feel faint or dizzy?		
5. Do you suffer pain or limited movement in any joint, caused by or aggravated by exercise?		
6. Are you taking any drugs or medication, or recuperating from a recent illness or operation?		
7. Are you pregnant?		
8. Are you unaccustomed to exercise and aged over fifty?		
9. Is there any other medical condition which may affect your ability to participate in sport?		

_____   _____
Signature   Date

Fitness Questionnaire (USA)

Regular physical activity is fun and healthy, and increasingly more people are starting to become more active every day. Being more active is very safe for most people. However, some people should check with their doctor before they start becoming much more physically active.

If you are planning to become much more physically active than you are now, start by answering the seven questions in the box below. If you are between the ages of fifteen and sixty-nine, the PAR-Q will tell you if you should check with your doctor before you start. If you are over sixty-nine years of age, and you are not used to being very active, check with your doctor.

Common sense is your best guide when you answer these questions. Please read the questions carefully and answer each one honestly: check YES or NO.

	Yes	No
1. Has your doctor ever said that you have a heart condition and that you should only do physical activity recommended by a doctor?		
2. Do you feel pain in your chest when you do physical activity?		
3. In the past month, have you had chest pain when you were not doing physical activity?		
4. Do you lose your balance because of dizziness or do you ever lose consciousness?		
5. Do you have a bone or joint problem that could be made worse by a change in your physical activity?		
6. Is your doctor currently prescribing drugs (for example, water pills) for your blood pressure or heart condition?		
7. Do you know of *any other reason* why you should not do physical activity?		

Talk with your doctor by phone or in person *before* you start becoming much more physically active or *before* you have a fitness appraisal. Tell your doctor about the PAR-Q and which questions you answered 'Yes'.

- You may be able to do any activity you want, as long as you start slowly and build up gradually. Or you may need to restrict your activities to those which are safe for you. Talk with your doctor about the kinds of activities you wish to participate in, and follow his/her advice
- Find out which community programmes are safe and helpful for you

Fitness Questionnaire contd.

If you answered 'No' honestly to all PAR-Q questions, you can be reasonably sure that you can:

■ start becoming much more physically active – begin slowly and build up gradually. This is the safest and easiest way to go
■ take part in a fitness appraisal – this is an excellent way to determine your basic fitness so that you can plan the best way for you to live actively. It is also highly recommended that you have your blood pressure evaluated. If your reading is over 144/94, talk with your doctor before becoming much more physically active

Delay becoming much more active:

■ if you are not feeling well because of a temporary illness such as a cold or a fever – wait until you feel better
■ if you are, or may be, pregnant – talk to your doctor before you start becoming more active

Please note: If your health changes so that you then answer 'Yes' to any of the above questions, tell your fitness or health professional. Ask whether you should change your physical activity plan.

_____   _____
Signature   Date

_____   _____
Signature of Parent   Witness

CHAPTER 11

NUTRITION FOR SPRINTING

by Dr Justin Roberts

As in many sports, nutrition is frequently overlooked when seeking performance improvements in sprinting. Whilst most athletes recognize the need to fuel training and recovery, nutritious wholefood meals frequently conflict with training demands so that when dealing with logistics and lifestyle many athletes resort to a rushed, 'quick-fix' solution involving processed foods and supplements.

Many world-class athletes pay less attention to their nutritional needs than to their training programmes, equipment, warm-up, stretching or mental preparation. Whilst many recognize that they are not eating appropriately, most believe that they eat 'healthily', although many athletes cite a variety of problems; these include:

- Feeling tired and lethargic before and during training
- Not feeling hungry in the morning (or too full before bed)
- Digestive problems – indigestion, bloating, over-fullness
- Experiencing mood swings, fluctuating energy levels, cravings
- Slow recovery between training sessions
- Running out of energy during training
- Fears over weight gains and/or digestive complaints (diarrhoea)

- Ignorance of the foods to eat for performance
- Ignorance of the effects and consequences of foods, nutrients and supplements
- Feeling stressed

The following dietary or nutritional issues are often reported by athletes:

- Not consuming enough calories to meet training demands
- Either skipping key meals or eating too late, often eating junk food or empty calories after training or competition
- Eating too fast and 'on the go'
- Craving certain foods, particularly sugary or savoury snacks
- Not consuming enough carbohydrate or protein following training sessions; increased needs for antioxidants and amino acids
- Not fuelling appropriately before or during training sessions
- Avoiding higher carbohydrate diets for fear of weight gain or digestive problems
- Eating generally low nutrient-dense foods after training
- Overloading on the wrong foods at certain times, or over-consumption of unnecessary supplementation concoctions

- Increased nutritional requirements, but not eating a variety of whole-food nutrients

THE IMPORTANCE OF NUTRITION

The link between training and performance lies with nutrition and recovery. Understanding recovery leads to enhanced adaptation and improved performance. Improved dietary intake is intricately linked to every bodily system (see Fig. 11.1). By eating a variety of wholefoods, and carefully assessing dietary habits, the athlete can improve digestion and metabolism, thus impacting on hormonal, muscular and cardiovascular physiology.

The quantity and quality of food consumed is important. Eating empty calories, highly refined or processed diets, lacking in nutrient variety, has negative consequences over time. Eating 'clean-and-lean' during training, and, to an extent, during competition, can improve an athlete. Clearly, athletes and coaches require a good knowledge of nutrition – which foods to eat and when to eat them.

Improvements in performance come from a managed approach to training and recovery, leading to an improved power-to-weight ratio (Tipton et al., 2007). Nutritional knowledge supporting health, training, recovery and competition is essential to a well rounded athlete.

Whilst a 'perfect diet' (whatever that is!) cannot, in itself, propel an athlete into world class, nutritional deficiencies and poor eating patterns (even during competition) can limit or reduce performance. Athletes and coaches should be mindful of *individual* nutrition approaches to optimize training

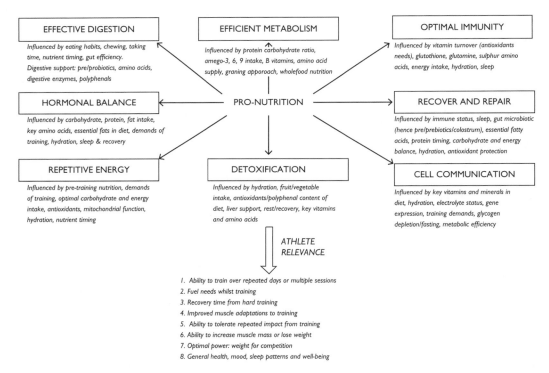

Fig. 11.1: **Why good pro-nutrition is important for sprinting events (with some examples).**

adaptations: whilst recommendations are made in this chapter, there is no one-size-fits-all approach.

When it comes to nutrition for sprinting there are several areas that need to be considered, particularly in the light of current research; these include:

- Nutrition for health
- Periodization of nutrition (based on training cycles)
- Nutrition for training (both fuelling needs and pre-training readiness)
- Nutrition during recovery (both short- and long-term)
- Nutrition for competition (especially when heats are only hours apart)

Generalized guidelines for all athletes are not the best way to optimize support. Individual needs, current intakes and lifestyle and training demands vary from athlete to athlete, and the principles here are better considered to be a starting point in tailoring an individual approach to nutrition. It is also recommended that athletes and coaches work with a qualified, professional nutritionist.

The nutritional programme should be 'built into' the athlete's training programme, and should focus on improving performance. From a behavioural change perspective, an aggressive approach to diet may detract from a training programme and alienate the athlete from good advice.

NUTRITION FOR TRAINING

Sprinters rely on the creatine phosphate and anaerobic glycolysis energy pathways that best meet the needs of the immediate and short-term bursts of energy that they undertake in training. This does not imply that they have lower energy needs than other athletes, and the indications are that many sprinters do not consume enough calories to meet their training needs. Guidelines stipulate that sprinters require 185–210kJ per kg^{-1} (of bodyweight) or (44–50kcal.kg^{-1}) (Manore et al., 2000). For an 80kg athlete this equates to 3,500–4,000kcals per day.

Athletes must recognize that their energy needs will be lower on rest days (2,200kcals per day) than on days of intense training (4,500kcals per day), and that they will need to consider varying their daily food intake to meet these varying demands, or calculate their average energy needs over a weekly period (that is, 2,800–3,500kcal per day).

Muscle glycogen, and hence carbohydrate intake, is a key factor in the ability to train repeatedly. Studies have shown that after just one resistance training session (Tesch et al., 1986; Creer et al., 2005) there was a reduction of around 20–30 per cent in muscle glycogen, and that after prolonged interval sprints there was a reduction of around 42 per cent (Krustrup et al., 2006; Spencer et al., 2005). The intake of carbohydrate prior to exercise has been shown to minimize the level of this reduction, which could impact on delayed fatigue and physical performance (Creer et al., 2005). As a result, sprinters should aim to take between 60–65 per cent of their total energy intake as carbohydrates.

Some experts recommend that athletes take 6g per kg^{-1} (of bodyweight) per day (Lambert et al., 2002), although this may be challenging for some. During intensive periods of strength and power training, between 5–7g.kg^{-1} may be required to maintain glycogen levels and allow for repeated training sessions. For an 80kg athlete this would equate to 400–560g of carbohydrate per day. During less intensive training, needs are likely to be lower – that is, 4–5g.kg^{-1} per day. Many sprinters frequently fall short of this.

TRAINING AND THE IMPORTANCE OF QUALITY CARBOHYDRATES

Many athletes are unaware of the difference between low and high glycaemic carbohydrates, and tend to eat highly refined, sugary or processed foods before training. Whilst muscles are particularly responsive to high glycaemic carbohydrates after training, some athletes may suffer negative consequences before training. Sprinters should aim to consume enough calories prior to training to meet their needs, but should also focus on easily digestible, lower GI foods.

Eating healthily should help to minimize gut discomfort or stomach cramps, and should avoid the rebound effects associated with increased insulin production. For some individuals, eating fast-releasing sugars such as sports drinks, sweets and energy bars within an hour of training can lead to 'rebound hypoglycaemia', where this food initially raises blood sugar, but then prompts a surge in insulin production which reduces energy levels and leads to lethargy and dizziness during training.

The solution is to have a pre-exercise meal between one and four hours before training. This meal should contain 1–4g of carbohydrate per kg of lean bodyweight. An 80kg athlete with 10 per cent bodyfat (or 72kg lean bodyweight) would therefore require 72–288g of carbohydrate. The meal should be based on low glycaemic foods with slow-release energy: for example, bran flakes or porridge oats with semi-skimmed milk, blueberries, or wholemeal toast for breakfast, and brown/basmati rice with chicken and peppers for lunch or dinner. Guidelines of 0.5g.kg^{-1} of liquid or easily digestible carbohydrates during training, particularly resistance sessions, have also been recommended (Slater *et al.*, 2011).

IMPROVING POWER-TO-WEIGHT RATIO – INCREASING MUSCLE MASS

During training, athletes aim to increase their power-to-weight ratios by reducing their bodyfat levels and maximizing lean muscle mass. As a result, the focus during heavy strength-training phases is often on utilizing nutrition to maximize muscle hypertrophy. When strength conditioning is then periodized with power-related sprint training, the intention is to use the training stimulus to improve sprint speed, and hence performance. Gaining muscle mass is largely influenced by energy intake as well as high quality protein levels. Simply consuming high levels of protein may not necessarily result in optimal gains, especially if total calories are comprised.

Focusing on gaining muscle needs to be undertaken as part of out-of-competition training, when it will not affect competitive performance. It requires the coach to determine the precise amount of muscle sought, and to regularly monitor the athlete's total bodyweight, lean bodyweight and bodyfat.

Simply introducing a new phase of strength training can result in dramatic muscle bulk gains due to anabolic hormone production, which may indicate a need to control, rather than increase, total calories or fat intake – that is, aiming for 2,500–3,000kcal.d^{-1} whilst maintaining relatively moderate protein intakes.

Whilst there is an indication that guidelines on protein intake should not be generalized due to many individual factors influencing protein needs, the consensus does suggest that sprinters should aim for 15–20 per cent of their energy intake as protein (for an athlete requiring 3,000kcal.d^{-1} this would equate to 450–600kcal from protein, or around 112–150g.d^{-1}). Most studies indicate that protein needs are often met by athletes, with sprinters probably requiring between 1.4–1.7g.kg-1.d^{-1} during regular training, and 1.7–2.2g.kg.d^{-1} during more intensive periods. For an 80kg athlete this would mean 136–176g of protein per day during intensive training.

There are two considerations to note at this stage: first, to reach this level of protein intake it may be better to consume small, regular meals over the course of the day – that is, between five to eight small meals centred around training. Nutrient timing has become an important aspect of performance nutrition, with studies demonstrating that protein intake around training (particular after hard training – see next section) can profoundly impact on muscle growth and its cross-sectional area, and power generation (Cribb *et al.*, 2006). The second consideration is that trained sprinters may require slightly less protein compared to novice sprinters; evidence suggests that during intensive training the body adapts by reducing protein turnover (Hartman *et al.*, 2006).

Whilst there does not appear to be any real harm in increasing protein intakes above 2g.kg^{-1} (unless there is an existing medical or kidney issue), the general contention is that high protein intake could be beneficial to meet energy requirements. The latest research indicates that combining training with higher protein intakes in power athletes may improve microbiota diversity (that is the type of bacteria we have in our gut), and support training adaptations (Clarke *et al.*, 2014).

Nutritional Keypoints for Increasing Weight/Muscle Gain

The following points are key for athletes seeking to increase weight/muscle gain:

- Increase intake by 500–1,000kcal.d^{-1} by increasing portion size as well as total carbohydrates (before fat or protein levels)
- When starting a resistance programme, assess the natural weight gains from training first; if necessary maintain the current caloric intake for the first six to eight weeks before increasing it
- Eat every two to three hours in order to minimize the potential negative effects of insulin production from larger meals, and to maximize natural anabolic hormone production
- During regular training increase protein to 1.5g.kg (lean mass)$^{-1}$.d^{-1}, and 2g.kg (lean mass)$^{-1}$.d^{-1} during harder training. Assess body composition ratios every week or two to modify dietary intake if needed. Eat quality proteins such as egg whites, turkey, beef, chicken, cod, tuna, salmon, cottage cheese, soya, quorn, beans and pulses. Try to eat as lean as possible if trying to reduce bodyfat at the same time
- If bodyweight increases are accompanied by increases in total bodyfat, this is an indication that calories are too high and/or the energy from saturated fats is too high, leading to weight gains from fat
- Aim to keep total fat to around 20 per cent of caloric needs: for a 3,500kcal diet, this would be around 700kcals from fat (or 77g – a range of 70–80g is often suggested: ~1g. kg^{-1}). Aim to keep saturated fat to around 10–15 per cent of total fat intake
- When caloric needs increase to, say, 4,500kcals per day, use meal replacements such as whey protein shakes and fruit-/milk-based smoothies with additional flaxseed/grounded seeds to increase calories, but never compromise on general nutrition intake. Eat a varied, wholefood, nutritious meal plan regularly
- Maintain fibre in the diet from vegetables and grains: dark green leafy vegetables,

brown/red/wild/basamati rice, porridge oats, quinoa as examples

■ Include a regular intake of foods high in essential fats (omega 3-6-9): salmon, tuna, mackerel, sunflower seeds, pumpkin seeds, olive oil, leafy greens – the use of omega fatty acids (4g daily as EPA and DHA) has been shown to increase testosterone production and support muscle gains (especially when combined with amino acids from proteins) (Smith et al., 2011)

RECOVERY: A SNAPSHOT OF THE SCIENCE OF MUSCLE GAIN

Recovery from training, with the associated muscle adaptations, is complex. Muscle protein gains (known as net synthesis) are a balance between protein use (or breakdown), and build up (or synthesize) over time in response to both heavy training demands, rest and nutritional intake. The balance of protein synthesis, particularly at the myofibrillar level (that is, the functional units of a muscle), tends to occur *following* a heavy training session. Current thinking is that muscle protein synthesis is delayed after heavy training due to elevations in enzymes (one in particular is AMPK). These enzymes increase due to reductions in ATP (very short-term energy stores) from training (Tipton et al., 2007). AMPK, for example, may act as a type of 'energy sensor' due to the metabolic and cellular stress caused by acute training.

In the short-term period after training this can lead to a net catabolic effect, whilst also limiting anabolic pathways including protein synthesis. This may be one reason why supplying essential amino acids in the recovery period may support faster recovery gains. It is also known that as the recovery period

continues, the influence of higher insulin levels in the blood may facilitate recovery. As a result, providing a combination of carbohydrates and amino acids may therefore support this process.

Although in the short-term recovery period enzymes such as AMPK may restrict protein synthesis, during the longer-term recovery period (in the hours after training) it is the activation of the mTORC1 pathway that appears to be important (Richter et al., 2009; Chen et al., 2003; Gibala et al., 2009). The mTORC1 (or 'mTOR' for short) pathway is one of the key mechanisms leading to protein synthesis. The latest scientific research indicates that a process of 'nutrient sensing' appears to take place in muscle during recovery through a number of signalling molecules (Rundqvist et al., 2013; Kimball et al., 2010; Kimball et al., 2006). The inclusion of carbohydrates, as well as essential amino acids (notably L-leucine), appears to be vital in allowing rapid signalling leading to faster protein synthesis gains (Coffey et al., 2011; Fujita et al., 2007; Drummond et al., 2008; Dreyer et al., 2008).

For the athlete, the message is that following bouts of hard training, a carbohydrate *and* a protein drink or snack may well support enhanced muscle recovery (Cribb et al., 2006). Key suggestions for nutrition during the recovery period include:

■ Within the first hour after intensive training aim to consume a carbohydrate/protein combination in the ratio of 4:1: that is, 60g of carbohydrate to 15g of protein. Most protein recovery formulas are close to this. Aim for 0.8–1g of carbohydrate.$kg^{-1}.hr^{-1}$ as a guideline. The use of liquid formulas – milk, banana, whey protein – is equally valid

■ Try to eat mostly lower glycaemic foods from two hours onwards (it is the total amount of carbohydrates that is important); however, some high GI foods are acceptable, for example a medium banana, cereal or a sports energy bar, a fruit yoghurt; a chicken sandwich and a medium serve of pasta

- Maintain hydration during this period – remember, fluid losses from sweating still occur post exercise; milk- and fruit juice-based drinks are just as useful as sports drinks/electrolyte solutions. The consensus is to be mindful of fluid lost during training, and to aim to minimize this deficit over a four- to six-hour period post training – so if the athlete has lost 1kg in weight from sweat losses, aim for 1.5–2ltr of fluid post training

- Try to avoid foods that may slow recovery or impact on further dehydration (especially during heavy training periods): caffeine, alcohol, high fat foods, fast foods, over-reliance on sweet foods. From observations, many athletes opt for 'quick fix' recovery foods (fried chicken, pizza, chips, take-away meals), particularly when training later in the day. Whilst 'treat' meals and rewards post-competition are acceptable, it has been noted that world-class performance is often the result of 'clean' eating during training

- Consider the inclusion of a 15–30g amino acid formula or lighter protein source – for example cottage cheese – about 30–45 minutes before bed. Research has indicated that the use of amino acids at this time may impact on net protein gains and recovery

IMPROVING POWER-TO-WEIGHT RATIO – DECREASING BODY FAT

For many sprinters, losing bodyfat is part of their muscle building and performance routines, with the impression that minimal bodyfat is vital for performance. This is not necessarily the case, however, and striving for very low bodyfat levels (<6 per cent) may encroach on 'essential fat' stores and have negative health consequences. At world-class level, bodyfat values of 4–10 per cent have been quoted.

The key point for the athlete is that maximum power-to-weight ratios relate to performance, but pushing for the lowest bodyfat level may also result in reductions in lean mass (hence a drop in power). As a result, athletes should have their body composition measured regularly, especially during pre-competition build-up periods so as to optimize power:weight. Focusing on increasing lean mass to above 90 per cent without reducing sprint performance should be a key aim.

Whilst training programmes often result in progressive reduction in bodyfat levels to an extent, there are some nutritional recommendations which can support this process:

- Reduce total fat intake on low volume training days or rest days to 20–25 per cent of dietary intake: thus for a 2,500kcal intake this would be 500–625kcal from fat (or 55–70g per day)

- Limit the intake of total saturated fats to <10 per cent of all fat intake (that is, 5–10g per day). For many sprinters this means being mindful to avoid eating highly refined foods, fast foods and take-away meals (for example fried chicken, crisps, cakes, biscuits, fries, pizza, burgers)

- Maintain a regular eating pattern: eat five to eight small meals per day, one meal every two to three hours, to improve metabolism. Aim for a subtle reduction in calories: 10–15 per cent from normal intake levels to minimize/avoid muscle loss. If muscle bulk is being aimed for as well, aim for a maintenance level or small increase in calories (5 per cent). It may be better to work with your coach on periodizing training with a rotation focus on increasing mass, then reducing fat in distinct cycles. Never compromise performance by trying to do too much

- Maintain a high protein intake: 1.5–2g.kg^{-1}, again eating small portions of protein with each meal: 20–30g every two to three hours
- Avoid being dehydrated – this does not mean overdrink, but having a 'graze' approach to fluid intake – sip on fluids 'little and often' (aiming for 2–3ltr per day, plus training needs)
- Don't drop carbohydrates too much, as this could affect recovery and training (try to have the majority of carbs from low GI sources). Instead, aim to have most of your carbohydrate needs in the morning, at breakfast and lunch. Eat 'low' in the evening: avoid refined sugars and starchy carbs in the evening (from, say, 5pm), and instead eat a high protein, vegetable-based dinner (salmon, two to three servings of vegetables), and minimize intake of potatoes, pasta, fries, rice and deserts at this time. This will impact on insulin function later in the day, leading to improved metabolism of fats over time
- Allow sufficient time to reduce bodyfat levels – crash reduction is not recommended as it can impact on performance. Instead aim for 0.5–1lb of fat reduction per week as a guideline
- Include essential fats in your diet (see section below)
- Consider the use of green tea extract (GTE) as part of your nutrient/supplemental intake. Green tea extracts (particularly caffeinated GTE containing ~400mg EGCG as an active component) have been shown to have the most productive effect on supporting increased fat oxidation (or use) during and following training (particularly aerobic base training). Whilst some other nutrients may be useful – for example L-carnitine, hydroxyl-citric acid (HCA) – these will not be discussed here as the evidence is often limited

The Importance of Essential Fatty Acids for Sprinters

Whilst potentially reducing total fat may support decreases in bodyfat, this should not be at the expense of the 'essential fats', particularly omega 3, 6 and 9. A multitude of studies now supports the beneficial effects of omega oils for athletes, including improvements in body composition and recovery from training. Such studies indicate that having 4g of omega-3 fatty acids (from EPA and DHA sources: oily fish, nuts, seeds, olive oil or supplemental) per day can support gradual gains in lean mass whilst resulting in reductions in bodyfat with training (Noreen et al., 2010).

In addition, as sprinting is associated with acute markers of stress or inflammation, sometimes resulting in muscle soreness, it is interesting to note that consuming 4g of omega-3 fats per day has been shown to reduce inflammation markers after intensive exercise (Bloomer et al., 2009). The message is clear: that omega-3 fatty acids should not be ignored.

NUTRITION DURING COMPETITION

One of the key issues faced by many sprinters is how to fuel during competition, as heats are frequently held in quick succession. Whilst the pre-training and recovery guidelines are useful – see previous sections – the following recommendations are key for sprinters during competition:

- Plan ahead, especially if travelling long distances. Travel can result in dehydration so avoid caffeine, alcohol and stimulant drinks as these can disrupt acclimatization post-journey and impact on pre-competition readiness
- Do not change dietary behaviour leading up to an event. There is generally no need to carbo-load in the ten to fourteen days leading into an event, but aim to maintain a normal-to-high carbohydrate intake
- On the day of competition aim for a meal about three to four hours before competition to permit digestion (Stellingwerff *et al.*, 2011). This meal should be carbohydrate biased, and might include for example ~80–350g (or 1–4g.kg^{-1}) of low GI carbohydrate egg, porridge oats, muesli, sweet potatoes, pasta, wild rice, spaghetti, pulses or beans, and contain a medium portion of protein, such as 20–30g egg whites, tuna, chicken, cod, beef, cottage cheese, whey
- Athletes should try to maintain hydration without over-consuming fluids fearing dehydration. Whilst athletes may be required to compete repeatedly during a day and be affected by fluctuating environmental conditions, simply maintaining a 'grazing' approach to fluid intake should offset any hydration issues. Aim to drink around 150–350ml of fluids (diluted squashes and fruit juices, electrolyte drinks, flavoured or natural water) after the pre-heat meal, but two to three hours before the heat
- Aim to maintain hydration by periodically sipping a dilute (2 per cent) sports drink up to 15min before the heat. This should help to maintain fluid levels and key electrolytes, especially in hot and humid conditions. Also minimize caffeine or stimulant drinks before competition: taking your usual coffee should not be an issue, but increasing to three to four coffees or stimulant drinks may lead to lethargy or 'rebound' after the first heat, and could induce subtle dehydration
- Prepare by taking any food, snack or drink that you use in training or for recovery, with you, in order to reduce your reliance on commercial facilities where resources may be limited
- For the duration of the competition avoid high-fat foods, fast foods, sweets or processed foods, as these may lead to gut problems, particularly during periods of stress
- Avoid sports drinks with a high level of fructose, which can increase digestive urgency in some people. Instead, plan for easily digestible foods such as bananas, apples, vegetable wraps, flapjacks, sandwiches/bagels, which are healthier and unlikely to cause issues before the next heat. If the second heat is within four hours, aim to eat a small snack (~30–50g carbohydrate) every hour or two, to maintain energy levels
- In line with the above point, between heats, aim to have an isotonic solution which can be sipped every 20–30min (2–4 per cent concentration, about 300–400ml per hour; little and often is frequently quoted for recommendations). For those who do not feel hungry in the mornings, try to include a portion of branched-chain amino acids with this drink
- Aim to stop eating around two hours prior to follow-up heats, but maintain a 'graze' approach to fluid intake

A WORD ON SUPPLEMENTS FOR SPRINTERS

Whilst supplementation (both clinical and sports specific) may offer bio-nutritional

POTENTIAL SPORTS SUPPLEMENTATION FOR SPRINTING

Supplementation	Guidelines for use	Reason
Creatine monohydrate (Casey et al., 2000; Cribb et al., 2007)	4 × 5g per day for 5–7 days to increase muscle levels; maintenance dose 3–5g per day for 6–12 weeks; cycle use during intensive training periods More useful in less trained individuals, vegetarian or vegan athletes Less useful in those with high initial levels of muscle creatine No evidence of reduced performance!	Improved use/turnover of creatine phosphate leading to shorter recovery time between sets. Improving training output leading to performance Note: can lead to increased water retention in early phases Combinations: with protein/ carbohydrate drink
Beta-alanine (Stout et al., 2006; Sale et al., 2010; Hill et al., 2007; Jones et al., 2002)	Loading dose: 3.2–6g per day in 4 divided dosages for approx. 4 weeks before intense training period Maintenance dose: 1.6–3.2g per day in two to four divided dosages during intensive training (6-week block) Adaptation effect sustained for approx. 8 weeks when supplementation period completed	Increases carnosine production, which may help buffer *intracellular* acidity during intense training allowing increased performance output Note: higher (>6g.d^{-1} or >10mg. kg^{-1}) or single (>0.8g) intakes can lead to paresthesia (flushing/tingling) sensations – hence loading phase of 3.2g.d^{-1} and maintenance of 1.6g.d^{-1} may be better for some individuals
Sodium bicarbonate (Tipton et al., 2007; Jones et al., 2002; Carr et al., 2011)	200–300mg.kg^{-1} <2hr before training – but 300mg.kg^{-1} or higher can lead to gut issues Potentially limited to events <1min in duration	Increases buffering capacity outside the muscle cells (extracellular) Needs to be practised in training to assess for effect or any gut issues
Caffeine (Davis et al., 2009; Goldstein et al., 2010)	3–6mg.kg^{-1} approximately 15–30min before exercise Note: >9mg.kg^{-1} may not offer improved benefits and values 9–13mg. kg^{-1} may begin to exceed maximum permitted level of 12µg.ml^{-1} urine – therefore be mindful of taking additional caffeine (stimulant drinks, coffee, tea) with anhydrous (powder) formulas*	Increases alertness, improves neuro-muscular fibre recruitment, improves reaction times Be mindful of potential 'drop off' effect if taken >60–90min before training, as can negatively impact performance Results may be better with non-caffeine users; could be useful to refrain from caffeine 2–4 weeks before competition

support, careful consideration should always be given to ensure that nothing consumed contravenes the World Anti-Doping Agency (WADA) List of Prohibited Substances (www. wada-ama.org). It is therefore prudent to consider carefully all substances prior to use.

There is little evidence that most supplements enhance *performance*, especially if a wholefood nutritional (and training) programme is followed; however, some products may be useful in supporting training adaptations that improve performance. These are outlined in the table, including possible mechanism and suggested dosage, and only relate to non-banned products which have been demonstrated to have 'ergogenic effects'.

* Sprinters should be mindful of *not* over-consuming commercial stimulant drinks which can have a short-term negative effect (headaches, lethargy, early fatigue, anxiety, withdrawal type effects) if consumed in moderately high quantities (> three drinks as example), particularly during competitive meetings and/or if combined with caffeine products.

SUMMARY

Nutritional practices for sprinters require a carefully tailored approach during progressive training and competition to meet the athletes' individual requirements. Essential consideration should be given to a variety of antioxidant-rich wholefoods, total carbohydrate intake to meet training demands, and higher protein requirement to support recovery adaptations. During competition, athletes should be mindful of minimizing foods/practices which may cause gastro-intestinal discomfort or reduce performance. Athletes (and coaches) are encouraged to work closely with nutritionists, especially with regard to the appropriate use of supplementation.

CHAPTER 12

DRUGS IN SPRINTING

by Wilf Paish, Tom McNab and Dr Geoffrey K. Platt

Part 1: Interview with Tom McNab

Q. When did you first become aware of drugs?

A. In 1964, at the Tokyo Olympic Games. Ron Pickering came back to me at our hotel to tell me that the Americans were being fed something called anabolic steroids at breakfast, only one in a long line of pills. This meant nothing much to me at the time.

(It is known that the Nazis undertook research on the effects of monkey glands on humans during World War II. It is suspected that the Eastern Europeans read the results of that research and may even have continued it after the war. GKP)

Q. But surely it was illegal?

A. At that time, IAAF rules on drugs consisted of only a few vague paragraphs, and it wasn't until 1973 that anabolic steroids were formally banned. By the late 1960s, a high percentage of international throwers were taking them.

(Although anabolic steroids were banned in 1973, there was no accepted test for them for a while, and then when the test was agreed, few competition tests were carried out and little out-of-competition testing was arranged for them, until around 1988. GKP)

A. And sprinters?

Q. I only really started to become aware of them because of the East German women competing against Andrea Lynch. They suddenly began to produce bulky women running in the low elevens. And earlier, prior to the 1968 Mexico Games, I had heard of massive back-to-back training sessions with the Americans at Lake Tahoe, sessions from which it would be impossible to recover. It therefore came as no great surprise to me that Bill Toomey ran 45.6 for 400m in decathlon, probably worth about 46.1 at ground level, which is still the fastest ever run in decathlon.

Q. What was the sequence of events in anabolic steroids with international governing bodies?

A. First to ignore them, or say that they didn't work.

(It is considered unethical to feed unnecessary medication just to undertake scientific research. The first research was conducted on old people confined to bed as they died of cancer. Anabolic steroids assist recovery after strenuous effort, so the initial research declared that anabolic steroids did not work. GKP)

Then came the ban and testing after 1973, but only in competition, the point when they were least likely to be detected. It was only post-Ben Johnson in 1988 that out-of-competition testing arrived. But behind everything was the elephant in the room, which was governing body involvement or complicity. This meant that the perpetrators were 'in' on every move by the international governing bodies, always ahead of the game.

Q. Involvement and complicity?

A. With the Communist nations there was direct involvement, with the capitalist nations there were varying degrees of complicity. We now know that the West Germans were not far off their East German neighbours, but the Americans varied between turning a blind eye and direct complicity. At Lake Tahoe prior to the 1984 Games their athletes were 'advised' by their sports scientists on how to avoid detection. And at least eight athletics 'positives' went missing at the Los Angeles Olympics. It's a sorry tale.

Q. Didn't the British Association of National Coaches make a formal statement about drugs after the 1972 Munich Olympics?

A. Yes – I wrote it! I issued a rather pious statement in 1973, saying that whatever the result, sport without ethics was not sport. And I proposed what was in essence the first cross-border testing programme.

Q. And the result?

A. Shock horror! Our International Athletes Club denounced it, and so did the governing bodies to a man. And I still have somewhere a Sir Humphrey letter from the Sports Council telling me that the Council of Europe had discussed drugs in sport, and the situation was therefore well in hand.

Q. Too early?

A. Yes, the time was not ripe. My 1973 statement was naïve, though in hindsight remarkably prescient, although the extent of

Communist-bloc programmes and the volume of drugs in the American system was not known by me at that point.

Q. And where are we now?

A. The World Anti-Doping Agency (WADA) has done some sterling work, but it must now be detached from direct governing body funding, and put under an independent organization such as the United Nations. Its funding should be massively increased, drawing mainly from the International Olympic Committee (IOC), who have surely a strong vested interest in clean sport. And it must now go far beyond testing, becoming much closer to an FBI-type operation. That means detective work, forensic activity, whistle-blowers, a whole proactive battery of skills, if we are ever to contain drugs.

(*The difficulty with this is that if WADA relies on government funding, then it will place itself in direct competition with the programmes confronting heroin and cocaine abuse, which are higher priorities. GKP*)

Q. I notice that you say 'contain'.

A. Advisedly. Drugs, like the poor, will always be with us. What we have to do is to make it more and more difficult to break the rules and get off with it. Had it been possible to offer Victor Conte a shorter sentence to come clean on the full extent of his activities, then American athletics might well have been dealt a near-mortal blow. And of course other sports much closer to American hearts, such as baseball and American football.

(*Victor Conte of the Bay Area Laboratory Company (BALCO) in California, USA, assisted the top American sprinters Tim Montgomery, Marion Jones and Kelli White, the top British sprinter Dwain Chambers, and Bill Romanowski the American footballer, with personalized cocktails of drugs. GKP*)

Because it is hardly a surprise that in a

nation in which almost a third of male teenagers have taken anabolics, their sport has been ridden with drugs since the 1960s. Hell, way back in the 1920s, their college coaches were already dosing their student-sportsmen with strychnine and caffeine, and injecting cocaine directly into muscles to get their injured footballers back on to the field.

Q. And here?

A. The evidence is understandably anecdotal. There is little mention of training drugs, but there is some talk of pre-competitive stimulants. But it would be wrong to be complacent.

Q. But surely we have encouraged foreign coaches with drug-backgrounds as athletes to lecture to our coaches, and even encouraged our athletes to be coached by them?

A. Yes, and at one point we even had the East German coach Wolfgang Arbeit primed to coach Denise Lewis! There has been an incredible naiveté here about the nature and worth of foreign coaches.

Q. But this surely goes well beyond drugs?

A. Yes. There has been the naive belief that 'somewhere over the rainbow' there was an untapped fountain of knowledge. Now this does not mean that at higher levels there are not marginal gains to be made from looking outside our borders. But the vast majority of our coaches are working in clubs with novices or teenagers, and so much of the information delivered to them was irrelevant.

Part 2: A Personal View of Drugs in Sport by Wilf Paish

Sport, *per se*, is a most healthy pastime. In the main, the abuse of performance-enhancing substances is limited to a very small proportion of elite performers, who stand to gain a significant amount either financially or politically. There is no doubt that success in sport is directly proportional to the amount of quality training that an 'athlete' is able to undergo, and still recover from in time to train again.

Hence in most cases, ergogenic aids are used to help the performer to recover from successive bouts of intense exercise, thus promoting an adaptation to the stressing agent. As a result of this desire to perform frequently at the highest possible level, the true cancer will always remain: the rich rewards that await those who are successful. We really do live in an era of the very wealthy elite performer, whose agent can demand whatever the market forces are prepared to pay.

This chapter will illustrate later that there is nothing new about people trying to enhance any aspect of their lives by taking advantage of what medical science, pharmacology, nutritional science and technology have to offer. Indeed, it is generally accepted that this is the only avenue available for progress. Specialized aspects of science are indicating to us more and more ways by which records can progress and old barriers can be broken down. Technology has given us improved footwear, carbon-fibre vaulting poles, tennis rackets, fishing rods and other appliances, as well as synthetic playing surfaces, aerodynamic projectiles, hydrodynamic sailing craft.

The list is almost endless. One has only to look at the restrictive, cumbersome clothing worn by soccer players fifty years ago, as depicted by photographs taken at the time, to see what progress has been made in sportswear alone. Where the evidence of progress could be instantly recognized, it was only a matter of time before other aspects of science, such as the pharmaceutical industry, would want to stake their claim to their share of the market.

Likewise it was just as logical that the health

food industry would also wish to capitalize on the potential of the 'performance-enhancing' market. The common links between the two industries, that of the pharmaceutical and health food industries, contribute much to the confused state as to what is, and what is not, a drug. While certain vitamins, minerals, proteins and enzymes are classed as foods, which can certainly enhance performance, abuse of such foods can prove toxic and can adversely affect the health of the abuser.

A number of the drugs found on the extensive list of banned substances, issued by the WADA, are essential for restoring the everyday health of many normal people. These include treatment prescriptions for such common ailments as asthma, migraine and IBS (irritable bowel syndrome), as well as medicines prescribed for such common ailments as colds and influenza, together with a number of other substances that are essential for restoring the health of many sick people.

While most of the doctors associated with doping control are quick to point out that there are almost identical substances that are not on the banned list, and which can be used as an alternative treatment, such an opinion is not shared by all doctors. Indeed, many doctors insist that the alternatives are not as effective and that sport is trying to adversely affect an honouring of the Hippocratic Oath.

In essence, this means that sport is discriminating against certain individuals. Indeed, if dope testing were fully implemented at all lawn bowling tournaments, a sport mainly considered to be the prerogative of those above middle age, most players would fail since they require beta blockers and certain anti-inflammatory drugs for the restoration of their normal health.

Perhaps the uncertainty as to what WADA considers to be legal and non-legal performance-enhancing substances stems from their inability to clearly define, or differentiate, between dope, drugs, medicines, health foods and all the other preparations that might fit into the vague term 'performance enhancers'.

However, I am convinced that the confusion arises mainly as a result of the dope testers' inability to illustrate that many of the substances on the banned list can significantly enhance performance. While I know that theoretically, pseudoephedrine could enhance performance through mental excitement, I have yet to read any valid research data which clearly indicates that this is fact. The same applies to a number of the other substances on the banned list: the assumptions made cannot be supported by sound research.

To date, I have never seen published any data relating to the reliability of the tests being used. It is generally accepted that there is no infallible scientific test, and there is always a tolerance factor stated to allow for both human and technical errors. This being an established scientific fact, how many of those tested either positive or negative come within the accepted level of errors? The only analogy that comes to mind is the fact that most civilized nations have abolished the death penalty for serious crime, and there has always been a strong lobby supporting the fact that several innocent people have lost their lives as a result of unreliable evidence.

The advent of dope testing has highlighted the diverse roles of the 'detective' and the 'criminal': that is, those people who are responsible for catching the person attempting to cheat the rules, and the person who is trying to avoid detection. While there is evidence to support the fact that the detection rate is increasing, it remains a fact that the 'criminal' is still several steps ahead of the 'police force'.

I cannot see a reversal of the roles until the testing procedures are changed. The truth is that only a percentage of pharmacological expertise is directed towards detection, while an equally large proportion is directed towards avoidance. The cheat is well versed in the use of blocking/masking agents, and is wealthy enough to invest in 'designer' drugs that stand every chance of remaining undetected.

As with so-called 'social' drugs, there has always been an illicit drug trade for those substances likely to enhance performance. The advent of dope testing has encouraged the establishment of a most lucrative clandestine industry, which claims to be able to provide anything at a price. Like all illicit dealings, the opportunity for abuse is widespread, and it has taken the provision of drugs away from the medical profession and placed it in the hands of the criminals.

There is already strong evidence of counterfeiting: the use of products designed for the veterinary trade, and the authenticity and purity level of many of the substances available, is causing the medical profession great concern. This situation is further highlighted by the current narcissus vogue, where many glossy magazines portray the well muscled man as an icon, so creating a social market for muscle-building hormones.

With the social drug scene and that involving sport performance enhancers now sharing much common ground, it seems hard to believe that there is likely to be a solution to the problem. Like the criminal, the sports cheat is highly motivated by the likely rewards available, at a risk, for those who will always attempt to ignore rules. However, the situation must never be allowed to become an excuse for indolence and for sacrificing ideals.

Most people closely involved with sport, and who also have a sound appreciation of the current situation, are aware that there must be a revision of the rules. However, a revision of the magnitude necessary to establish fairness can only be implemented by a group of well informed people who are prepared to start with a 'clean slate'. Furthermore any system so devised must then be adequately

policed, with a punishment that will act as a permanent deterrent.

A close examination of current doping policy forces one to question the motives that influence the underpinning philosophy. It would appear that the rationale is one of policing rules so that cheats can be identified, and also one of protecting the health of both current and future generations of competitors. But on both counts the scheme falls miserably.

As far as the letter is concerned, it encourages competitors to resort to drugs where detection is unlikely, such as the various derivatives of growth hormone, thus encouraging a possible end result which could be acromegaly – a giant that literally splits out of its skin. It also encourages them to use cocktails of different drugs in order to avoid detection or to minimize side effects, where the complete interaction of the chemicals is unknown. This is all far removed from the situation where a group of well qualified doctors will use drugs to restore health.

As for catching the cheats, even those intimately involved with the detection process realize that many escape detection, and there are those who believe that the process is more directed towards 'punishing the naughty boy'! Most elite sportsmen and women regard themselves as professional entertainers.

It is well recognized that many entertainers use performance-enhancing substances to help them satisfy their audiences. Indeed, a number openly flaunt the rules of the land. Long-running television programmes such as *Top of the Pops* and the various song contests make us aware that there is an element of competition involved, mainly linked to record labels and royalties.

Most people involved in the administration of sport – that is, its political wing – fail to recognize the analogy with the 'pop star'. They remain influenced by the dated *mens sana in corpore sano* (sound mind in a sound body) philosophy, that all of those who participate in sport are the most ethical, law-abiding citizens. Yet in competition, those same people have been known to deliberately kick or bite an opponent. Perhaps the Battle of Waterloo was won on the playing fields of Eton, but the Gulf War certainly was not.

Many philosophers in sport recognize that in the modern world, sport might have taken over from war. With such a philosophy, where in the rankings of legitimacy, in times of war, between a sniper's bullet and an atomic bomb, might a few anabolic steroids be placed? Perhaps an extreme view? Nevertheless, one only has to spend a short while in the company of very highly motivated sportspeople to realize there is little for them to recognize, that will stop them from achieving their goal.

Can the rules of sport, certainly off the field of play, be any different from those laws which govern society as a whole? Those laws which are the responsibility of the judicial system? There is already evidence, from those lawyers supporting their athlete clients, that they believe that the logical hypothesis is correct and that the laws of the land are final. Perhaps the outcome of Modahl vs. British Athletics or Ben Johnson vs. Athletics Canada and the IAAF might well determine the future.

The sport and leisure industry is one of the fastest growing economies of the world. With computers, machines and the like undertaking many of the chores previously performed by people, it was only a matter of time before there was a massive reduction in the workforce necessary to run the economy, thus providing people with more leisure time. For many, this has given them the opportunity to participate in a wide variety of leisure pursuits. 'Leisure wear' is now the 'vogue' uniform of the public at large, and trainers have become the 'vogue' footwear, so much so that a normal pair of lace-up shoes looks out of place, and tracksuits have certainly taken over from jeans as the common casual wear.

In basic terms these are now all products of what was once a sports' clothing and footwear industry. The new industry is keen to promote its past relationship with sport, creating the sporting icon for their advertisement campaigns, bringing with it lucrative endorsement contracts – which means that yet more financial pressures will be placed on the shoulders of the elite performer since all the sponsors will be anything but philanthropists and will be demanding their 'pound of flesh'.

For many, this increase in leisure time has provided the opportunity to spectate, whether it be direct through the turnstiles of a stadium, or via the ever-increasing opportunity provided by television. As a result the ultimate is created, that of the spectator believing that he is in part ownership, in which situation he can determine the level of entertainment he is prepared to accept.

If the product is wrong, the spectator will show his concern by reduced gate receipts or viewing figures. Such a situation brings with it a demand from the players always to perform at the level of expectancy determined by the spectator. Demands of this nature can do little else but encourage the use of performance-enhancing substances.

An increase in leisure time does not always bring with it an enhanced lifestyle: instead it has created the era of the 'couch potato' - the person who will sit and watch all that television has to offer. The medical profession rapidly became aware that this was adversely affecting the health of the population.

Since to a degree this situation was created by the media itself, the propaganda machine, attempting to encourage a healthier lifestyle, soon started to have an effect. Participation in marathons, jogging, aerobic classes, 'step' sessions, together with a whole host of movement-based activities, have brought with it a new clientele, with massive spending power, providing the industry with a greater revenue with which to attract its icons.

Changes in our patterns of work have brought with it massive changes in the way society reacts and behaves. It is inevitable that, associated with these changes, will come changes in our values, a change in our former code of ethics, a situation which is well reflected in our appreciation of sport. The age of the internet has brought with it a freer and better-informed society. Indeed, the person determined to cheat the rules of sport needs look no further than the internet, since many of the banned substances are openly advertised and readily available. Perhaps many will accept that this is the price of freedom.

Fortunately, at the time of writing, the leaders of sport are beginning to recognize the need of a policy review. Juan Antonio Samaranch, the former President of the IOC, attracted media attention over his widely condemned views which appeared in the Spanish newspaper *El Mundo* in late July 1998. Apparently he shared a belief that drugs which do not damage one's health should be legalized in sport. Only a passing reference to 'performance enhancement' was made. The debate was further escalated by the intervention of Primo Nebiolo, the President of the IAAF, the most powerful body within the IOC, who was swift to support his colleague in a crisis.

Only a total review will be acceptable. The rules governing the use of performance-enhancing substances have evolved in a most haphazard way. Once a substance has been detected in the urine sample of an athlete, it has usually been supported by legislation to ban the substance. The action has always been one for expediency rather than one of an informed delay – a delay to examine whether or not the substance found sufficiently enhances a performance to warrant a ban. Moreover it has been made without there

being a consideration as to whether or not a valid test can be formulated to assess the presence of the substance in a urine sample, and whether or not the system can be policed.

The current situation has led to abuse and confusion, as witnessed in the 1998 Tour de France cycle race. It would appear that in this case the action was taken by the local police force, acting on a tip-off that certain riders/ doctors/coaches had in their possession illegal drugs, and not through any doping control enforced by the race promoters.

In this chapter I have tried to highlight most of the contentious issues relating to this very emotive topic. For many, the very future of sport rests with the ability of the controllers of sport to introduce and police a fair policy successfully. Indeed the whole ethos of sport is at stake. The significance of these issues will be more fully debated at intervals throughout the text.

The aim of this chapter is essentially educational and not prescriptive. The information compiled is the result of almost half a century of being involved in international sport. For a large part of this time I have been an informed observer of the doping-in-sport scene and an avid collector of relevant data. As an observer with an interest in the scientific research involved and at the same time a person close enough to the 'sharp edge' of sport, I understand intimately all the physiological, psychological and sociological implications.

Though not a person involved in the politics of sport, I am, nevertheless, one who has a strong desire to eliminate discrimination and to shed hypocrisy; a person committed to a belief that it is important to pass on to the next generation a situation better than the one inherited. This can only be achieved by better education, and by more and more people becoming aware of the truth and who will, hopefully, be in a position to influence the policy makers.

CHAPTER 13

MENTAL SKILLS TRAINING IN SPRINTING

by Dr Andrew Cruickshank, Susan Giblin and Professor Dave Collins

In previous chapters, a detailed picture has been painted of what peak performance in sprinting looks and feels like. This has included ways in which it can be achieved through coaching and conditioning, and with physiological, biomechanical, analytical and lifestyle support. In this section we take up the baton and look at the mental factors behind peak performance. In doing this, we identify some of the most important mental qualities and skills that help athletes prepare for competition and to perform when it matters most.

We begin by presenting a model that we have used to help athletes to develop and deliver on their abilities. We then consider some key mental skills that help athletes to best use this model. After this we look at planning and organization, covering processes that can be engaged on competition day. In the last section we describe some mental skills that can be applied from the warm-up all the way to crossing the finishing line (or handing over the baton). Like sprinting itself, we cover our ground quickly and, hopefully, successfully!

PROMOTING PEAK PERFORMANCE – A GUIDING MODEL

Our model for guiding peak sprinting performance is provided in Fig. 13.1. As shown, its structure is made up of three major parts: *components, plan* and *execution*.

This model is based on the idea that peak performance relies on an athlete having the 'right' attributes, combined together in the 'right' plan, and delivered with the 'right' execution. Although we say 'right', it is important to remember that there is no single 'correct' set of attributes, plan or execution strategy. Rather, each of these is shaped by the unique physical, technical, tactical and mental attributes of each athlete (as well as their competitive level and goals). The exact nature of this individual 'blend' may also vary from race to race, and will definitely evolve throughout an athlete's career.

Similar to performance profiling (Jones *et al.*, 1993), identifying and working on the factors that help to deliver peak performances provides athletes with a model against

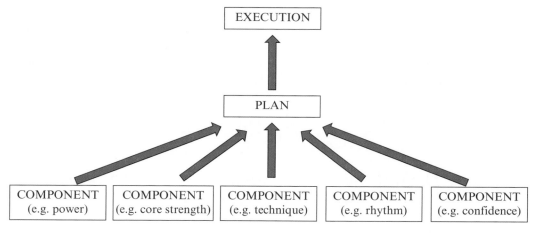

Fig. 13.1: The 'components-plan-execute' model of peak performance.

which their training can be compared and evaluated. This approach also encourages a *process* orientation, one in which the athlete recognizes and works on the things that *lead to* them running as quickly as possible. This is especially useful when there are no key events on the horizon and therefore no 'competitive buzz' to harness.

As events approach, particularly important ones, the identified components are then packaged into a specific plan for the event's specific conditions (for example indoors/outdoors; domestic/international) and demands (for example the need to achieve qualification times; the presence of rivals). Finally, this plan is then delivered through a well rehearsed execution strategy, which is again designed for the specific contexts of specific races.

Before addressing the planning and execution phases of the model in more detail, we now identify some core psychological skills which help to develop, consolidate and refine the components of peak performance.

OPTIMIZING THE COMPONENTS OF PEAK PERFORMANCE

While identifying the components of peak performance is important, athlete success largely depends on core mental skills. Indeed, excellence most often comes from goal setting, planning and organization, commitment, focus and distraction control, imagery, coping with pressure, quality practice, self-awareness, self-regulation, grit, resilience, seeking and using support networks, and realistic performance reviews (Collins *et al.*, 2012; Duckworth *et al.*, 2007; MacNamara *et al.*, 2010a; MacNamara *et al.*, 2010b; Macnamara *et al.*, 2011; Toering *et al.*, 2009). As athlete development is based on a cycle of 'target–plan–do–review', we focus here on goal setting.

Important for creating, focusing and sustaining motivation (Locke *et al.*, 1984; Locke *et al.*, 1985; Locke *et al.*, 1996), we are yet to meet any athlete (or human!) who does not use goal setting to at least some degree (for example 'I want to win the next race'). Less common, however, is the expert use of this technique. Specifically, best practice depends on a detailed consideration of the nature, content and packaging of goals.

The Nature of Goals

In terms of their nature, goals can be divided into three types which can be used on their own, but ideally in combination. These three types are process goals, performance goals and outcome goals (Filby *et al.*, 1999; (Hardy *et al.*, 1996).

Process goals: These goals relate to the process of performance – in short, the factors required to perform a task at a desired (and realistic) level. These goals encourage a focus on the task at hand, motivation to do the task well (rather than the outcome of winning), required behaviours, and appraisal against the task or one's prior performance on the task. As an example, a common process goal in sprinting may be to improve the explosiveness of one's start out of the blocks.

Performance goals: These goals relate to performance on a task. They are useful for directing focus towards required behaviours, or to enhancing competitiveness (either against either one's personal bests, or other athletes). Continuing our example above, a common performance goal for an athlete seeking to improve his or her starts may be to work towards hitting 10m in a specific time.

Outcome goals: These goals relate to the outcome of performance – in short, the result achieved. Motivation from this type of goal is usually based upon winning or beating others. Outcome goals are arguably the most magnetic of all, and it takes good discipline to remain focused on the process of performing on the day; in short, to stay focused on what you need to do, as opposed to what it might be like if you won. Continuing with our prior example, an outcome goal for an athlete working on their starts may be to reach the first 10m ahead of his or her training partners or the known performance of others.

Given their different implications, each type of goal is useful for one purpose or another; the trick is knowing which goals to set for which purposes, when, and in what combination.

The Content of Goals

Although the content of goals (that is, what they focus on) will depend on the particular task or objective, athletes and their coaches/support teams would also do well to follow the SMART (Weinberg *et al.*, 2003) or SMARTER principle. This means that as much as possible, goals should ideally be **s**pecific, **m**easurable, **a**djustable (or **a**greed with coach/support team), **r**ealistic, **t**ime-locked, **e**xciting and **r**ewarding.

However, as many athletes often want more than they have got and to do it better than they have done before, a handy 'bolt-on' is setting 'multi-level' goals. So, if a realistic target is one that the athlete should be hitting roughly 70 per cent of the time, then this is taken as a 'level one' goal: achieving this would be 'good' and show that progress had been made. Pat on the back! To account for the 'I want for more' factor, a 'level two' target would then reflect a level that the athlete may have a 40 per cent chance of achieving (equalling a 'great' effort).

Finally, a 'level three' target may then be one that the athlete has a 10 per cent chance of hitting (equalling a '*how phenomenal was that?!*'). In this way, athletes can recognize different levels of success and can make an effort to really push beyond their limits (which are often self-imposed).

155

The Packaging of Goals

Finally, expert goal setting also requires targets to be packaged effectively. One of the most effective ways of achieving this, in our experience at least, is through the application of a 'nested' approach (Abraham et al., 2011; Martindale et al., 2005; Martindale et al., 2012). As shown in Fig. 13.2, this involves setting short-term targets (for example, daily/weekly goals) which are nested within medium-term targets (for example, multi-month training blocks). These medium-term targets are then nested within long-term targets (for example, extending over the length of a full season/ multiple seasons).

This structure therefore helps athletes to engage with day-to-day activities that support their medium- and long-term goals (and vice versa: see the feed-forward/feed-back loops in Fig. 13.2). It also helps to keep athletes adaptable, focused on process, and continually working towards (and not against!) the 'bigger picture'. For example, an outcome goal of 'I want to win my next big race' can be helpfully shaped into 'if I want to win this major race in four years, then I'll probably have to finish in the top three at that race in six months if I'm going to be on track.'

PLANNING FOR PEAK PERFORMANCE 'ON THE DAY'

As peak events get closer, attention should start to move away from how components may be improved, towards how they can be packaged into the best plan for race day. Indeed, while it is tempting to 'tinker' (that is, to try and make things as 'perfect' as possible), there is a point where athletes need to accept and build confidence in 'the cards they've got'. Hopefully this is a strong hand, but if it is not,

too much tinkering close to the event will make it even worse!

Similarly, the best plans are created well in advance of race day so they do not distract the athlete during final training phases, yet are kept open enough for finer details to be included when event schedules and conditions become known.

We now consider how planning at 'macro' and 'micro' levels can support peak performance on the day.

Macro-Level Planning: Race-Day Planners

Race-day plans have three key core roles: to set out exactly what the athlete is going to/ has to do before competing; to reinforce the athlete's strengths/confidence; and to prevent (or minimize) 'noise' from potential disruptions. Indeed, although it may seem impossible that an athlete could arrive at a major event without an important bit of kit, this can and does happen! As the pressure of competition can ignite even the most fireproof of situations, things that have never been noticed or gone wrong before must be treated as possible disruptors (Collins et al., 2014; Wilson et al., 2011).

By anticipating various situations and developing strategies to deal with them, race-day plans therefore help to avoid the challenges and errors of 'thinking under pressure' when unexpected events are faced in competition (for example, a delayed start time).

On these principles, the race-day planner in Fig. 13.3 includes key primary behaviours (that is, obvious functional tasks), coping behaviours (planned responses to challenges) and outcomes (what the athlete wants to be thinking/feeling at different stages) (Rushall et al., 1987). Also included are other important preparation behaviours

Levels of Focus	Goals			
	Year 1	Year 2	Year 3	Year 4
Long-term Outcome Goals	Level 1: Top 10 at World Champs Level 2: Finalist in World Champs Level 3: Top 6 at World Champs	Level 1: Finalist at Commonwealths Level 2: Top 6 at Commonwealths Level 3: Top 5 at Commonwealths	Level 1: Finalist at World Champs Level 2: Top 5 at World Champs Level 3: Medal at Worls Champs	Level 1: Top 6 at Olympics Level 2: Top 4 at Olympics Level 3: Medal at Olympics
Medium-term Performance and Process Goals	Phase 1 (Winter Training/Initiation of Changes) [Defined goals here]	Phase 2 (Indoor Events/Test and Refine Changes) *Example 3-level performance goals:* achieve average of sub-1.95/1.90/1.85 seconds for first 10m; achieve average of sub-6.60/6.55/6.50 seconds for 60m *Example process goals:* continue to refine explosiveness of starts through integrated conditioning, biomechanics, nutrition, and psychology support, test/refine pre-performance routine to facilitate optimal pre-race confidence	Phase 3 (Start of Outdoor Season-Consolidated Changes) [Defined goals here]	Phase 4 (Mid-End of Season-Deliver Peak Performances) [Defined goals here]

	Weeks 1–2	Weeks 3–4	Weeks 5–6	Weeks 7–8
Short-term Performance and Process Goals	[Specific performance/process goals based on training/competition plan]	[Specific performance/process goals based on training/competition plan]	[Specific performance/process goals based on training/competition plan]	[Specific performance/process goals based on training/competition plan]

= feed-forward and feed-back loops between nested levels   = feed-forward and feed-back loops within nested levels

Fig. 13.2: An outline representation of 'nested' goal setting.

Timeline	Physical Activites (What I'm doing)	Mental Activities (What I'm thinking/feeling)
Wakening-Up to Departing for Venue	- Wake-up call, open curtains - Check hydration and start/adjust appropriate fluid intake - Shower - Check forecasted weather conditons - Check kit and prepare/pack snacks and fluid against checklist - Brief walk and stretch to loosen up (within hotel if cold/wet) - Breakfast (follow nutrition/hydration strategy) - General chat with support team/watch news on TV/avoid social media - Return to room and collect items 30 minutes before departure time - Make way to meeting point 15 minutes before departure time	*Guiding Phrase: 'Relaxed and prepared'* - Ease myself into the day/loosen up
Travelling to Venue	- Ensure leg space in vehicle - Listen to the radio/music - Avoid social media	*Guiding Phrase: 'I know what I need to do'* - Start to gradually switch on - 1 x run through arriving at venue and coping with media attention and interactions with/distractions from competitors (imagery) - 1 x run through pre-performance routine/race (imagery)
Arriving at Venue to Starting Warm-up	- Register, receive heat/lane draw, confirm timings - Find spot to set up base (not too close to holding area or competitors to enable segmented preparation and prevent distractions) - Walk/get a look at track and get a feel for the conditions - If start time already delayed, go for a brief walk and find somewhere to sit away from venue/central area (depending on length of delay, make any necessary minor adjustments to pre-performance routine with coach/support staff, run through imagery of routine and race, listen to music, play games on tablet device)	*Guiding Phrase: 'Complete my set-up'* - Jobs done - Get comfortable with surroundings - (Re-)Familiarise with venue and protocols *Guiding Phrase: 'Tick over and stay ready'* - Ease back on mental intensity

Fig. 13.3: Competition preparation strategy (as based on Rushall and Potpeter, 1987, and Wilson and Richards, 2011).

(for example, mental rehearsal). Please note that this planner relates to preparation for the first race of a day, or a day when there is only one race.

Planning for multiple heats over multiple days will clearly require an extension of this outline, and the inclusion of more strategic components (for example tactics, such as laying down an early marker or slipping under the radar to set up a big impact in the semis/final). A planner for use ahead of a relay would also include team-oriented content.

By setting out physical and mental activities against specific time slots, this planner encourages a sense of control, reduced/manageable anxiety, and protects against avoidable errors. Importantly, all of these outcomes help athletes to get into, and then stay in their *individual zone of optimal functioning* (Hanin et al, 2007) (that is, when they experience an optimum mix of emotions).

By ensuring that the content of this plan is led by the athlete and includes key guiding phrases, this can also frame self-talk during the build-up to an event. This tool also helps athletes to evaluate the *full* process of their performance on the day (as well as the race outcome itself) and therefore supports long-term development.

By setting out physical and mental activities against specific time slots, this planner encourages a sense of control, reduced/manageable anxiety, and protects against avoidable errors. In addition, by ensuring that the content of the plan is led by the athlete and includes key guiding phrases, this can also frame self-talk in the lead-up to an event. Importantly, all these outcomes help athletes to get into, and then stay in, their *individual zone of optimal functioning* (Hanin, 2007) (that is, when they experience an optimum mix of emotions). It should be noted that Fig. 13.3 can also act as a template for the race-day planners of coaches and other support team members. More specifically, any individual involved at the event can use this to detail their own schedule, and the behaviours, thoughts and emotions that allow them to perform at their own peak.

In addition, these planners are often best developed with the help of others. In the case of the athlete, for example, input should be sourced from the coach(es) and any other relevant members of the support team (for example, physiotherapist, psychologist). This open discussion can help to make sure that all areas are considered, as well as optimize team-level involvement and commitment. Importantly, all of these features can optimize the athlete's feelings of control, support and confidence in the lead-up to race day, as well as on the day itself. By having a shared understanding of the ideal preparation for the athlete, these plans can further help to keep all members of the team on the same page – which is especially handy in the 'white heat' of competition where distractions are plentiful.

By its nature, the race-day planner encourages a focus on the *process* of performance rather than its potential outcomes. However, although these plans are highly detailed and include apparently obvious activities (for example, packing snacks and fluid before departure to the venue), this does not mean that they should be rigidly adhered to if this is not required. Indeed, the race-day planner might be most successfully used as a 'check and balance' tool, allowing for a level of adaptability and improvization to deal with any truly unexpected events (that is, those which have not been prepared for). That said, some athletes will benefit from adhering tightly to this plan. As with any skill or technique, using the planner as a reminder, or more as a strict guide, should be based on the individual's needs and preferences.

Over the long term, developing and using race-day planners for *every* event increases the chances that beneficial behaviours will be engaged before competing. More specifically, as the planner provides a reminder to use behaviours that optimize preparation and ultimate performance, which are then reinforced by the consequent feelings of control and confidence, athletes are more likely to use these at the next event. Indeed, if these race-day planners are consistently applied, individuals will soon recognize when they are missing! Importantly, by seeing the athlete feel comfortable and confident, these outcomes are then also likely to be experienced by the coach and other support team members.

Finally, the race-day planner can also be used to help athletes (and others) evaluate the full process of their performance on the day (as well as the race outcome itself). As part of a thorough review that supports long-term development, focus should centre on the plan's success in preparing the individual, as well as its usefulness for dealing with the expected *and* unexpected challenges of competition. This process can then lead on to the continued refinement of race day planners for the future.

Micro-Level Planning: Pre-Performance Routines

Having developed a plan for managing the broad period before an event, another more detailed plan can then be used from beginning a warm-up right up to the firing of the starting gun. Indeed, while peak performance requires the seamless transfer of skills from training (Singer *et al.*, 2002), the perceived pressure to perform often gets in the way of this process as the event nears. In this way, developing and using a pre-performance routine (PPR) can be a reliable way to get (and stay) physically and mentally switched on.

Used to create a sense of control and to prime the athlete's neuromuscular system during physical warm-up (Lam *et al.*, 2009), PPRs relate to behaviours, emotions and thoughts (Cohn *et al*, 1990). As one example, the 'PPR Funnel' that we have used with athletes is shown in Fig. 13.4. While the timing and content will vary across athletes and events, the outline shows how mental and physical processes can promote a focus on the task, appropriate arousal and confidence. A trigger is used to initiate the athlete's entry into the funnel (for example, a certain time before the race start) and then further triggers are used to prompt progress through each phase (for example, walking out on to the track).

As the PPR picks things up where the race-day planner left off, athletes are therefore aware of what they should be doing at all times before the race and (hopefully) feel in control and confident. PPRs can also play a key role when athletes are faced with unexpected events. For example, an athlete can adapt their PPR to handle delays in the call room or false start situations – we discuss this in more detail later. For now, it should be noted that back-up planning should be included when developing a PPR (as shown in Fig. 13.4).

Of course, athletes in relay events will need to adapt their routines to include team-based processes (for example team communication, baton practice). Although the routine of the first leg runner may not vary much from that used for their individual events, the rest of the team must prepare themselves for additional challenges – again, more on this later. For the moment, and as a particularly effective aspect of preparation, we now discuss pre-performance imagery.

IMAGERY

As imagery engages the same areas of the brain that are used in real experience, this

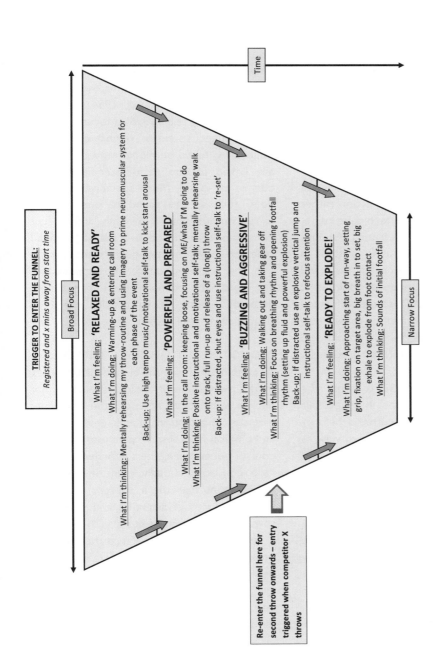

Fig. 13.4: The 'pre-performance routine funnel'.

skill can be applied to warming up for a task without physically doing it (Holmes *et al.*, 2001). In this way, athletes should include visual, auditory, emotional, environmental and kinaesthetic information to enhance the vividness and impact of the produced images (Holmes *et al.*, 2001).

For example, athletes can imagine themselves walking confidently on to the track, feeding off the noise from the crowd, getting set in the blocks, anticipating and then hearing the starting gun, exploding from the blocks, hearing their foot-fall, forcefully exhaling, pumping their arms and legs, lifting their head and fixing their gaze on a point beyond the finish, and powering through the line.

In terms of movement, athletes are advised to rehearse their *full* sprinting action rather than individual parts of their technique immediately before racing. Indeed, such routines are best conducted with 'real rhythm' in 'real time' to replicate the actual flow and duration of peak performance (Holmes *et al.*, 2001). Imagery should also be performed under similar physical conditions to real performance; for example, when warming-up starts in full race kit and with a raised heart rate.

It should also be relative to what the athlete can deliver (so not imaging skills that they have never demonstrated before). Imaging performance from one's own view, as if watching oneself on television, or a combination of both, can be effective depending on the individual needs of the athlete and the purpose of the imagery.

As well as warming up movement, imagery also plays a key role in mood regulation and motivation, outcomes that are especially useful for coping with the uncontrollable and unexpected features of competition. For example, when heat and lane draws are made, the athlete could add this information to their imagery routine and produce a more specific

rehearsal of their race plan (as deployed during their PPR). Imagining oneself coping with the challenges of the call room can also help athletes to maintain focus, manage arousal levels, and promote confidence when space to engage in physical warm-up is limited.

PROMOTING OPTIMAL RHYTHM

As well learned skills often break down when efforts are made to explicitly monitor them (that is, move right leg like this, then left arm like that) (Baumeister *et al.*, 1984; Masters *et al.*, 1992; Hardy *et al.*, 1996), a focus on kinesthetics, speed, sound or rhythm encourages athletes to focus on global movements that are linked to top performance (MacPherson *et al.*, 2008). More specifically, 'holistic cues' such as the sound of one's footfall can promote optimal rhythm and reduce conscious control and overthinking. Indeed, research shows that pre-performance strategies that include holistic, movement-based cue words (for example 'bang') can promote automatic and efficient skill execution (MacPherson *et al.*, 2009).

PROMOTING AUTOMATIC CONTROL

As athletes approach the blocks and take their marks, the volume of thinking should further decline with focus now on the final cues that sustain attentional focus, emotional set, and physical readiness. To promote automatic control (when racing feels effortless, involves little conscious thought, and time flies) it is important that these triggers encourage a narrow focus of attention and direct this towards race-relevant factors.

As an example, one useful strategy involves the athlete fixing his or her gaze on a point beyond the finish line (known as the 'quiet eye') (Vickers *et al.*, 1996). This technique has been associated with decreased conscious thought and extended subconscious processing of the task at hand (Vickers *et al.*, 2007). In addition, auditory triggers also play an important role in helping athletes to react to the starter's orders.

For example, an athlete could focus on their breathing rhythm until called to their marks by the starter. At this point the athlete could respond by performing a few vertical jumps, and then deeply inhaling and exhaling before settling into their blocks. On hearing 'set', the athlete focuses on taking a sharp intake of breath and then forcefully exhaling when the starter's gun is fired.

While this normally marks the end of a PPR and the start of the execution, in other cases problems are presented by false starting (either by the athlete themself or their competitors). Given the chance of this occurring (or any other distraction), a 'secondary PPR' or recovery mechanism can help to manage the increased pressure to control reactions in the second start, prevent over-hesitation, and channel the adrenalin derived from the initial start.

For this, a combination of instructional self-talk (that is, telling yourself what to do) and behavioural triggers can be used to regain control and then to guide re-entry into the original PPR funnel at the correct stage. For example, on experiencing a false start an athlete may:

- Use self-talk to self-instruct and reframe the situation: 'OK – relax and go again. Nothing's changed' (*conducted on the walk back from the stopping point on the track back to the blocks*)
- Visually fixate on their blocks to avoid any distractions from other athletes/to maintain their focus on the job (*used on the walk back from the stopping point on the track back to the blocks*)
- Use their passing of their blocks on the walk back as a trigger to check for any unwanted physiological and mental tension

– a big exhale of breath at this point to 're-set'
- Use self-talk to re-enter the final phase of the main PPR and get into its rhythm ('re-enter and rhythm')

Clearly, the content of this secondary routine will depend on each athlete. Additional self-talk that offers self-assurance and reinforcement may also be required if it was the athlete who false started rather than another competitor.

In-Race Processes

To protect (or recover) automatic execution during a race, a focus on something in the external environment is usually more beneficial for skilled athletes than a focus on internal states (for example, fatigue) or technical elements (for example, arm positioning). As such, athletes are often best also to focus on auditory cues during the stages of a race to prevent their thoughts from interfering with automatic execution, such as footfall or respiratory rhythms.

If auditory cues are difficult to sustain due to noise from the crowd, a single cue word that replicates rhythmic or holistic aspects of performance can be used to initiate or regain control (for example 'ping, ping, ping' to represent short, snappy ground contact time).

In terms of relays, self-talk and visual and auditory cues can also be used to support take-off and communicate baton transfer. For example, athletes may fix their gaze on a point at the start of the change-over zone and repeat 'wait, wait' until they see their teammate's foot strike this point. This focus also works to limit distractions posed by incoming athletes and/or the team's race position.

The athlete then begins to accelerate, focusing his or her attention on forcefully exhaling until he or she hears the command 'hand' from their team-mate. On receiving the baton, the athlete then fixes his or her gaze on the top bend of the track and repeats 'boom, boom, boom' to replicate the rhythm of powerful cadence when accelerating.

CONCLUDING COMMENTS

We hope that this chapter has illustrated some important mental factors and processes for peak performance in sprinting. Against our components-plan-execute model, we have paid particular attention to expert goal setting. In doing so, we have discussed how a 'multi-level' and 'nested' approach can enhance motivation and help athletes to continually work towards their 'bigger picture'. We then focused on planning/preparation, and ways in which athletes can get in the best mental (and physical) shape possible when they take their marks, and then to the finish as quickly as possible.

Self-regulation, attentional control, emotional patterning, mental rehearsal, rhythm and automatic control were all identified as particularly important for this process. As noted throughout, the precise way in which all of the presented factors are addressed or used *will* vary from one individual to the next. Indeed, an approach which one athlete finds effective may be one that has an almost opposite impact on another.

As such, we encourage any athlete or coach who has found our contribution useful (or hopefully parts of it, at least!) to carefully explore, experiment with, and continually refine these principles and tools. May they bring much speed!

CHAPTER 14

THE INCIDENCE AND TREATMENT OF INJURIES IN SPRINTING

by Dr Gino di Matteo

Running is a sport that presents a significant risk of injury to the participant, the nature of which will vary depending on the sub-discipline being undertaken. While distance athletes typically suffer from over-use pathologies (the accumulation of multiple event micro-trauma to tissues), the sprinter, in his or her quest for the development of explosive power, has a greater vulnerability to single-event macro trauma, more likely leading to the sudden failure of contributing muscles, tendons and joint structures.

Invariably, the occurrence of injury is as a result of one or more contributory factors that combine, each of which may be identified as a primary cause or a secondary contributor. These factors can be further sub-divided into intrinsic factors (such as muscular inadequacy, imbalances, flexibility) or extrinsic factors (such as shoes, surfaces).

Clear and accurate identification of these factors is imperative for injury prevention or management, and the collective responsibility for this lies with all members of the team – the technical and strength and conditioning coaches, the supervising clinician/ physiotherapist, the rehabilitator and, most importantly, the athlete. The use of motion analysis and movement screens has become increasingly popular for the assessment and identification of faulty movement patterns, and these tools have been recommended to help prevent injuries in athletes (Dallinga, Benjaminse and Lemmink, 2012).

Due to the very nature of sprinting and sprint training, athletes are continually at risk of sudden catastrophic failure of musculoskeletal structures. Although not unheard of in sprinters, over-use injuries are more common in the distance athlete. The following is not meant to be an exhaustive list of pathologies seen in sprinters, but rather to present common injuries that the sprinter may encounter, and to provide an indication of management, rehabilitation and prevention strategies that athletes, coaches and clinicians may consider.

POSTERIOR THIGH PAIN AND INJURY

The posterior thigh is a common site of problems for athletes, though the assumption is often that all posterior thigh pain is as a result of hamstring tears. However, other structures in the posterior thigh include sciatic nerve and the conjoint hamstring tendon, and referred pain into the posterior thigh from the back or hip is also a relatively common finding.

Hamstring Tears and Tendinopathy

The hamstrings are a group of three bi-articular, fusiform muscles situated in the posterior compartment of the thigh. They collectively attach above the hip joint to the ischial tuberosity of the pelvis, with the biceps femoris having a second proximal attachment to the posterior aspect of the lower half of the linea aspera of the femur. Distally, they attach below the knee to the tibia (semimembranosus and semitendinosus) and the fibula head (biceps femoris). See Fig. 14.1.

Hamstring tears are by far the most prevalent pathology encountered by sprinters, and have a higher incidence of recurrence than any other injury (Hoskins and Pollard, 2005b), with biceps femoris being the most commonly affected muscle (due to the asymmetrical length of the two heads, with each head being controlled by different portions of the sciatic nerve).

The hamstrings are brought into action throughout the majority of the running gait cycle (Clanton and Coupe, 1998). They assist the gluteal muscles with the extension movement of the hip through the stance phase (acting initially concentrically, then eccentrically), and contract concentrically in the early swing phase as the leg is lifted off the ground (Yu et al., 2008). During the terminal part of the swing phase they are expected to produce high forces, sufficient to control the extension moment produced by the quadriceps. It is at this phase and during this type of contraction that the hamstrings are most vulnerable (Scache, Dorn, Blanch, Brown and Pandy, 2012; Scache, Wrigley, Baker and Pandy, 2009).

Contributory factors to injury have included imbalance between the strength/

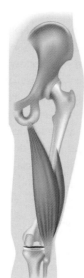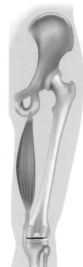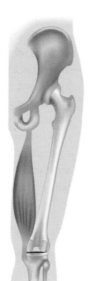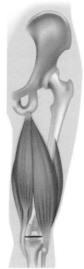

Fig. 14.1: The hamstring muscles. (Shutterstock)

Biceps femoris   Semitendinosus   Semimembranosus

endurance of the quadriceps and hamstrings themselves. This can lead to overload injury as the hamstring is attempting to control the quadriceps extension moment (Yeung, Suen and Yeung, 2009).

Tightness can also contribute to failure, as inadequate length of these muscles can lead to overstretch injury as the hip is thrust into flexion while the knee is continuing to extend (Daneshjoo, Rahnama, Mokhtar and Yusof, 2013). In addition, and possibly most importantly, poor hamstring eccentric control has been shown to be a significant factor when looking at injury, as it can lead to asynchronous firing of the muscles and therefore an uneven distribution of forces (Stanton and Purdham, 1989)

Hamstring tears can range from minor muscle pulls (grade 1), to tendon degeneration or failure (tendinopathies or tendon rupture/avulsion) or gross failure on one or more muscles (grade 2 partial tears, or grade 3 complete rupture). The athlete will often identify a specific injury point, invariably pulling up suddenly in pain and unable to complete an event. Immediate management should follow standard first-aid procedures of PRICE (protection, rest, ice, compression and elevation).

Ignoring injury and attempting to continue with high-load activity can cause a relatively minor tear to develop into a higher-grade injury, lengthening forced abstention from sport and further increasing the risk of re-injury. The early use of non-steroidal anti-inflammatory agents has been questioned in this type of injury, as inflammation is an important part of the healing process, especially in the primary phase of repair (Clanton and Coupe, 1998).

Immediate examination may seem rather unremarkable, with the athlete complaining of only mild discomfort on stressing the injured muscle/tendon. Re-examination twenty-four to forty-eight hours later may better reveal the full extent of the injury, with the subject having difficulty walking, let alone running, as a result of bruising (evident in higher-grade tears) and referred pain due to the intimate relationship of the hamstrings with the sciatic nerve (Aggen and Reuteman, 2010).

The management of hamstring injuries has long been a contentious subject. The lack of high-quality research has failed to provide any degree of consensus, with most opinion being somewhat anecdotal. However, most clinicians would agree that treatment includes a period of relative rest (usually seven to ten days) with the promotion of healing achieved by the use of ice, compression, electrotherapeutic modalities such as ultrasound, interferential or shock-wave therapy (Cacchio et al, 2011), and soft-tissue work such as massage and myofascial techniques.

Subsequent rehabilitation must focus on regaining the strength and flexibility of the injured muscles in a controlled manner. Late-stage rehabilitation must include eccentric control and specificity of training, with some authors proposing specific hamstring regimes that mimic their function during sprinting – for example, HamSprint drills (Cameron, Adams, Maher and Mission, 2009) or Nordic Hamstring exercises (Copland, Tipton and Fields, 2009).

Since previous hamstring pathology is the best predictor of injury, prevention is always going to be favourable. Focusing on hamstring strength, flexibility and control, and the identification of risk factors by the use of various screening procedures in early athletic careers, can be most useful in protecting the individual from injury (Hoskins and Pollard, 2005a, 2005b).

Return to sport is dependent on the grade and site of injury. Typically muscle injuries do heal well as the tissue is vascular and repairs quickly, while tendinopathies typically are slower at healing due to poorer blood supply. Recovery rates can range anywhere from two weeks – low-grade injury (Kilcoyne, Dickens, Keblish, Rue and Chronister, 2011) – to fifty weeks (high-grade and tendon injury).

Sciatic Nerve Tension

A common complication of hamstring injury includes involvement of the sciatic nerve. This may be a primary injury of the nerve (damage of the nerve at the time of injury) or secondary (involvement of the sciatic in the reparative process leading to neural adherence to the surrounding muscles). It is often difficult to differentiate sciatic nerve tension from hamstring injury. Some authors have proposed including neural mobility exercises prophylactically to prevent further complications (Aggen and Reuteman, 2010).

Neural mobility issues involving the sciatic nerve are a relatively common finding and are often misdiagnosed as hamstring injuries (Puranen and Orava, 1988). Early differentiation is important, and the use of imaging techniques such as diagnostic ultrasound or magnetic resonance imaging, can help with accurate diagnosis (Carillon and Cohen, 2007) and avoid unnecessary and inaccurate clinical management.

ANTERIOR THIGH, EXTENSOR MECHANISM AND LATERAL KNEE PAIN AND INJURY

Although tears of the quadricep muscles are far less common than hamstring injuries, they are nevertheless seen in sprinters. However, pathologies of the associated extensor mechanism (the patella, quadriceps tendon and patella tendon and associated structures) are more commonly encountered by clinicians.

Quadriceps Tears

The quadriceps is a group of four muscles situated in the anterior of the thigh. The three vasti (medialis, intermedius and lateralis) are single joint muscles and their organization is such that non-traumatic injury of these muscles is very unusual. Rectus femoris is the only quadricep muscle that crosses two joints (hip and knee), which predisposes the muscle to strains higher up the leg. However, the bi-pennate structure of the muscle is such that loads are distributed over a wider area, providing some degree of protection. All four muscles converge to form the quadriceps tendon attaching into the tibial tuberosity and containing the patella. (See Fig. 14.2)

Although not exclusively, injury to the quadriceps is far more common in sports that require repetitive kicking than sprinting in isolation (Mendiguchia, Alentorn-Geli, Idoate and Myer, 2013).

Anterior Knee Pain and the Extensor Mechanism

Anterior knee pain is a global term used to describe a collection of pathologies in the front of the knee. These may be from the patella, the patella tendon, Hoffa's fat pad or any of the bursae (fluid-filled sacs in the anterior aspect of the knee).

PATELLO-FEMORAL JOINT

The patello-femoral joint is a synovial joint between the posterior surface of the patella and the anterior surface of the lower end of the femur. The patella is expected to track

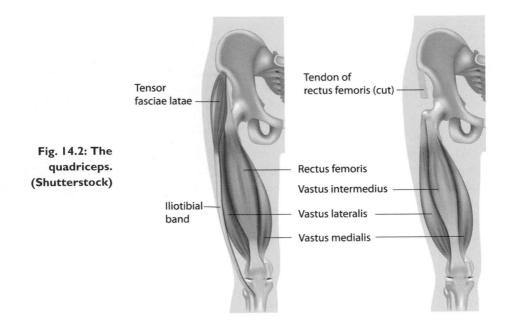

Fig. 14.2: The quadriceps. (Shutterstock)

up and down in the groove on the front of the femur in a very specific direction as the knee moves through flexion and extension. A poorly tracking patella can lead to soften-ing and fissuring of the joint cartilage on the posterior surface, and eventually cause pain in activities that involve loading the knee in a flexed position.

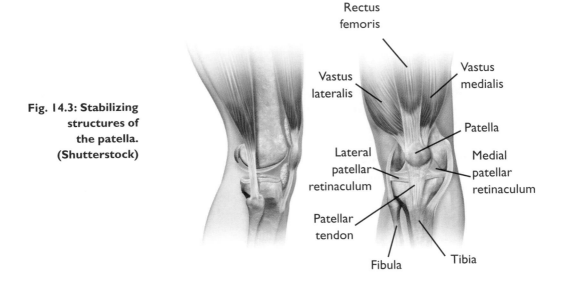

Fig. 14.3: Stabilizing structures of the patella. (Shutterstock)

Maltracking of the patella can come about as a result of a number of mechanical factors. Imbalances between the lateral and medial (vastus lateralis and medialis) quadricep muscles can cause the patella to move laterally in its groove – synergistic imbalance. In particular, inadequacy of the lower fibres of vastus medialis (vastus medialis obliquus (VMO)) have been implicated. This particular portion of muscle has been shown to be very susceptible to the inhibitory effects of knee pathology and swelling, and it is usually the first part of the quadriceps to demonstrate atrophy (Palmieri-Smith, Kreinbrink, Ashton-Miller and Wojtys, 2007).

Clinical management focuses on improving the contribution from this muscle by performing targeted exercise (such as knee extension in the final 30 degrees of movement), or adductor exercises with particular focus on adductor magnus (this muscle provides attachment to some of the superficial fibres on vastus medialis, and increasing the tone of the adductors will provide it with a more stable base from which it can work).

In addition, poor functional limb alignment can result from inadequate gluteal control from above, which in turn can lead to a lateral tendency of the patella (McConnell, 2002). Simple movement screens – for example, observing movement of the knee during a squat or a lunge – can identify this. Ideally this should be seen to move over the second toe, but in athletes with poor gluteal control or imbalances, the knee is seen to drift medially. This is managed by re-educating gluteal control with appropriate rehabilitation exercises such as clams and bridging.

The use of proprioceptive taping to further stimulate the gluteal muscles during activity is becoming increasingly popular and an effective tool in re-educating gluteal control.

Even with good muscle control, patella maltracking can result, if the passive restraints on

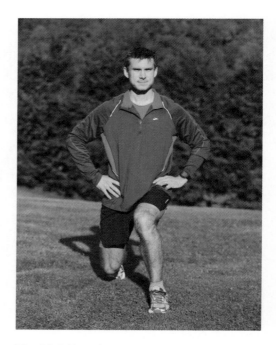

Fig. 14.4: Poor knee movement during the lunge.

the lateral side of the patella are shortened. Patella motion is guided by the patella retinculae (thickenings in the anterior capsule) and the anterior portion of the ilio-tibial tract (a fascial thickening in the lateral thigh).

Ensuring adequate relative mobility of these structures can be achieved by joint mobilization, with particular attention needed to release the lateral retinaculum and the ilio-tibial tract (by means of stretching, foam roller and soft tissue work).

Finally, when considering patella-femoral tracking, one must also look at the overall mechanics from the foot up. An excessively pronated foot, or a foot that fails to re-supinate during propulsion, can lead to forces that cause the lower limb to remain in internal rotation. This causes the patella to track laterally and to maintain uneven pressure in the patella groove on the front of the lower femur (McConnell, 2002). (See Fig. 14.5.)

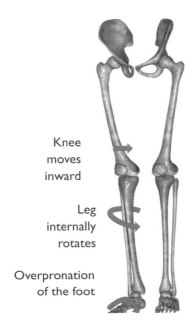

Knee moves inward

Leg internally rotates

Overpronation of the foot

Fig. 14.5: Overpronation leading to internal lower limb rotation and lateral tracking of the patella. (Shutterstock)

The correction of foot mechanics can be achieved by checking footwear and using suitably posted orthotics and/or corrective exercises.

The uses of a variety of patella taping techniques have become increasingly popular in the management of patella tracking problems. Whilst taping techniques such as McConnell taping have been used in an attempt to provide a mechanical restraint to patella motion, Kinesio taping techniques (Fig. 14.6) have recently become more commonplace. This type of taping is a low-load taping method that has the effect of providing a sensory (proprioceptive) stimulus, which has the effect of altering muscle function and therefore dynamic tracking.

Fig. 14.6: Kinesio taping. (Photo: Shutterstock)

PATELLAR TENDINOPATHY

Although the patella tendon is an inherently strong and well organized structure, pathology is not uncommon in athletes who perform high-load activities. More common in jumpers than sprinters (hence it is often referred to as 'Jumper's Knee'), it is typically a degenerative change that occurs most commonly at the inferior pole of the patella. It is worth a mention because the site and nature of the pain that the athlete presents with, is similar to that of patella-femoral joint pathology.

A combination of poor blood supply, and extremely high stresses that pass through the patella tendon, makes this a difficult pathology to overcome. Histological studies have shown this to be a degenerative pathology rather than an inflammatory one, therefore the term 'tendinosis' (rather than tendinitis) is more appropriate. Furthermore, an anti-inflammatory management strategy will have only limited effect, and more modern regimes

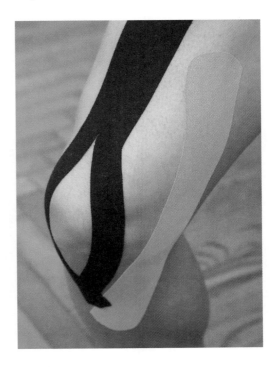

have shifted the focus towards stimulating tissue re-growth and protection (for example friction massage, ultrasound, eccentric quadriceps exercises such as squats on a decline board, and focus on the shock-absorbing characteristics of the training shoe) (Peers and Lysens, 2005).

FAT-PAD IMPINGEMENT AND BURSITIS

Hoffa's fat pad is situated under the patella tendon immediately above the deep infrapatella bursa (see Fig. 14.7). Impingement of either of these structures can occur by hyperextension of the tibio-femoral joint, or by compression of the lower patella against the femur. These structures give a disproportionate degree of pain considering the amount of tissue damage. This is due to the high number of pain nerve endings in these tissues. However, due to their vascular nature both of these structures respond well to conservative treatment (ice, rest, ultrasound), taping to offload the fat pad, and anti-inflammatory agents (Dragoo, Johnson and McConnell, 2012).

Lateral Knee Pain

The most common structure to be affected in runners is the lower part of the iliotibial band (ITB). This is a broad fascial thickening passing from the hip, and extending down to the lateral aspect of the knee. At the lower end it is separated from the lateral femur by a pouch of fluid known as the iliotibial band bursa.

As the knee flexes and extends, the ITB rolls back and forth over the lateral aspect of the lower femur and, if tight, can cause excessive compression and irritation of the bursa – this is known as iliotibial band friction syndrome (ITBFS) and can be extremely painful and disabling. (See Fig. 14.8.) Contributory factors include poor stabilization at the hip from the gluteal muscles, and excessive pronation or relative tightness of the ITB itself. It is more common in longer-distance runners (400m and up), but short-distance sprinters can develop it in longer training session or when doing hill work.

Management is aimed at controlling the inflammation – this can be achieved by

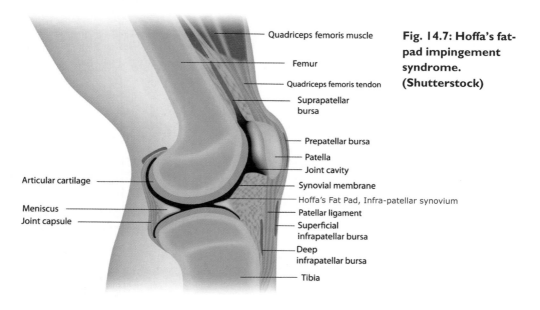

Quadriceps femoris muscle

Femur

Quadriceps femoris tendon

Suprapatellar bursa

Prepatellar bursa

Patella

Joint cavity

Synovial membrane

Hoffa's Fat Pad, Infra-patellar synovium

Patellar ligament

Superficial infrapatellar bursa

Deep infrapatellar bursa

Tibia

Articular cartilage

Meniscus

Joint capsule

Fig. 14.7: Hoffa's fat-pad impingement syndrome. (Shutterstock)

LOWER LEG AND FOOT PAIN AND INJURY

Injuries in the lower leg region generally fall into one of a number of categories – the first is sudden failure, or recurrent failure, of muscle and/or tendon, the most common of which is a tear of the calf complex, and more specifically the superficial calf muscle, the gastrocnemius.

Secondly, stress fractures can occur at specific sites due to recurrent abnormal load, faulty lower limb biomechanics, and nutritional or hormonal deficits.

Finally, there is a collection of pathologies that are often grouped together under the category of 'exercise-related lower leg pain'. These include the ubiquitous 'shin splints', compartment syndrome and medial tibial stress syndrome.

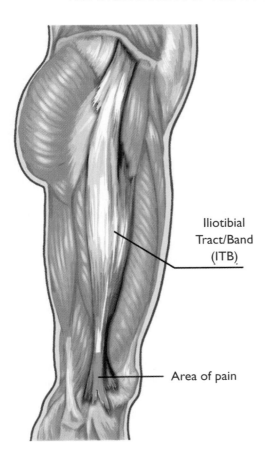

Iliotibial Tract/Band (ITB)

Area of pain

Fig. 14.8: Iliotibial band friction syndrome. (Shutterstock)

conservative management such as ice and ultrasound, with the use of non-steroidal anti-inflammatory agents, or, in persistent cases, by means of hydrocortisone injection (Ellis, Hing and Reid, 2007). It is important to address contributory factors such as foot mechanics and posture, muscle imbalances, in particular of synergistic groups, and achieving mobility of the ITB itself.

Calf Tear and Achilles Tendinopathy

The calf complex is divided into two compartments: the deep compartment containing the muscles tibialis posterior, flexor digitorum longus and flexor halluces longus, and the superficial posterior compartment. The superficial compartment contains three muscles that are the main drivers of the foot during dynamic gait activities.

Gastrocnemius: A bicipital muscle that arises from the posterior and lateral surfaces of the femur and forms the superficial part of the Achilles tendon. Typically classified as the explosive component of the calf and therefore well developed in the sprinter.

Soleus: Lies deep to the gastrocnemius and arises from the posterior surface of the tibia, fibula and interosseous membrane. It passes down to form the deeper layers of the Achilles tendon, and is typically the more postural or endurance component of the calf.

Plantaris: A small muscle that arises from the postero-lateral surface of the lateral condyle of the femur, and passes down to attach into the Achilles tendon or occasionally directly into the calcaneum (the heel bone).

Calf tears in sprinters most commonly occur (although not exclusively) in the gastrocnemius, as this is the muscle that is utilized forcefully, in particular in the initial propulsive phase out of the starting blocks. The medial head is more susceptible than the lateral head, and this is often due to faulty foot biomechanics, as excessive pronation generates more tension on the medial tissues than the lateral tissues.

Although calf tears can be severely disabling, they do respond well to conservative management. Early ice, compression and relative rest is imperative, and any modality that promotes healing (ultrasound, massage, ice, laser) will significantly speed up a return to sport. However, it is important to ensure the calf regains full concentric and eccentric strength as well as flexibility.

Furthermore, imbalances of the plantarflexors can lead to the overload of any one muscle. The group are synergists and all contribute to plantarflexion. The failure of one muscle to contribute to the overall movement can lead to domination by another muscle. In the management of calf injuries the clinician should consider an even distribution of force.

Other possible sites of lower leg injury that may arise due to high forces generated, in particular at the start of a race, are pathologies of the Achilles tendon. Structural malalignments due to faulty foot posture, muscular imbal-

ances or degeneration in the older athlete can all lead to recurrent stress and irritation of the tendon. In rare occasions, rupture can occur – this is often as a result of a devitalized or unhealthy tendon in athletes who have chosen to ignore warning signs of swelling, heat or pain arising from the Achilles region. While muscle injuries in the calf do respond well to conservative management, the Achilles tendon is more resistant due to the high concentration of forces passing through it, and the inherently poor blood supply that is often noted in such dense structures.

A number of management strategies have been proposed for Achilles tendinopathy. The consensus is that there is actually relatively little, if any, inflammation present (Alfredson and Lorentzon, 2000), but that it is a failed healing response to the normal micro-failure that occurs during exercise (Longo, Ronga and Maffulli, 2009; Wilder and Sethi, 2004). The cumulative effect eventually leads to a tendinosis (a degeneration of the tendon), which although still utilized as a form of clinical management, remains resistant to traditional treatment with anti-inflammatories and rest.

Instead, clinicians are turning to more aggressive forms of treatment that aim to create stress on the tendon to promote earlier fibrosis and repair – for example loaded or single leg eccentric calf raises, cross frictions, stripping of the tendon sheath or dry needling (Fahlstrom, Jonsson, Lorentzon and Alfredson, 2003; Longo et al, 2009). Poor success rates and a generalized lack of consensus for optimal management for Achilles tendon pathology may lead to more drastic measures in the management of this condition, such as prolonged immobilization with the use of plaster or Aircast® boots, or even surgical options such as stripping of the tendon sheath, ultrasound guided scraping of the tendon, debridement of the tendon sheath, or even tenotomy (Alfredson, 2011; Maquirriain, 2013)

Exercise-Related Lower Leg Pain, Shin Splints and Tibial Stress Fractures

All sections of the limbs are divided into separate compartments by fascial sheets (intermuscular septa), each containing a functional muscle group: for example in the thigh we have the anterior (quadriceps), posterior (hamstring) and medial (adductor) compartments. The compartments of the lower leg are no different, the only slight variation being the fascial sleeves that cover each functional group, which are denser and tighter.

This has the effect of improving venous return back to the heart by maintaining pressure on the deep vessels. However, as a result of the increased metabolic demands placed on muscles during activity, increased blood flow can lead to increased intra-compartment pressure, which in turn can cause a number of potential pathologies.

Firstly, changes in the intra-compartmental pressure can cause blood vessels within the compartment to become overly compressed. The loss of blood flow leads to ischaemic changes, which can at best cause discomfort in the shin or calf during exercise that clears on rest, or at worst can cause avascular necrosis of the tissues the vessels supply. In extreme cases surgical fasciotomy is indicated, where the compartment pressure is released by surgical splitting of the deep fascia. More minor cases can be treated conservatively and managed by soft tissue mobilization, stretching the myofascial tissue with foam rollers, massage and so on.

Biomechanical mal-alignment of the foot and lower leg can cause uneven tension through the deep fascia, and irritation of its insertion point along the medial tibia or anterior tibia can cause a periosteal (the fibrous covering of the bone) reaction, which, if left untreated, can eventually lead to tibial stress fractures. Conservative management with the use of orthotics and strengthening local muscles to hold foot alignment in the correct position (for example, inversion exercises), or the re-education of more proximal muscles such as the gluteal muscles, can help offload the fascia sufficiently to alleviate symptoms.

It is important to note that although athletes will present once they have started to complain of symptoms, the very nature of sport and training does lead to tissue damage that for the most part is sub-clinical. The normal reparative capacity of the body stops this from becoming symptomatic. When the cumulative effect of this tissue damage and degeneration outstrips the natural healing process, we see over-use injury.

Whilst factors such as faulty biomechanics and anatomical anomalies can be identified as obvious contributors, less obvious factors such as changes in volume or intensity of training, nutritional or hormonal deficits, and low bone density (especially in women who have had menstrual cycle disturbances or amenorrhea for periods longer than six months) coupled with the stresses of sport, can lead to typical pathologies such as tendinopathies or stress fractures.

Tendinopathies can be managed successfully by the use of soft tissue mobilization, biomechanical correction, addressing muscle imbalances and promotion of healing (Wilder and Sethi, 2004). In the same way as other tendons are slow responders, those around the foot and ankle similarly require long periods of modifying training and periods of abstaining from competition.

The identification of stress fractures can only be confirmed by radiological examination

(X-ray, CT, MRI or radioactive isotope bone scan), and management must include immobilization, relative rest and extended periods of abstention from sport. If found deficient, nutritional aspects must be addressed by the supervising physician and/or nutritionist – for example low calcium intake, excessive alcohol, caffeine or smoking. Common sites of stress fracture include the tibia, fibula (less common), the calcaneus and the metatarsals, although other areas can also be affected (Wilder and Sethi, 2004).

SUMMARY

Sprinting is a high load but high reward sport. Athletes are always striving to achieve better times in their own particular event, and consequently are pushing their body to the physical limit. There is a very fine dividing line between being at peak physical condition and being injured. Whilst the pathologies and contributory factors presented above are a summary of common injuries and causes, this is by no means a complete list.

Sprinters in particular, as a result of their diversity of power training, will most commonly injure muscles (in particular hamstrings and calves) due to overload, but can also develop problems in other areas of the body (back, upper limb and other sites in the lower limb). Early assessment and immediate management by a suitably qualified professional will reduce the time needed to return to sport, and accurate identification of contributory factors will allow implementation of a suitable prevention strategy.

CHAPTER 15

PERFORMANCE LIFESTYLE FOR SPRINTING

By Dr Geoffrey K. Platt

As soon as a young person decides to commit to becoming an elite athlete, then he or she must give serious consideration to his or her lifestyle. Time spent working in a gymnasium, sports hall or track will be wasted if the athlete fails to get enough rest, eats the wrong food, abuses cigarettes, alcohol or drugs, is worrying about his or her financial situation, or regularly misses appointments. Elite sport is a twenty-four-hour a day commitment, each and every day, for between ten and twenty years.

A young athlete soon realizes that success in sport is not just a blend of technical and tactical skills and physical and mental qualities, and that in order to maximize performance, he or she must consider his or her personal lifestyle, and understand the ways in which this will affect performance during practice and competition.

It should be noted that, like many other terms, 'performance lifestyle' has been hijacked by the English Institute of Sport (EIS) to cover its activities, and allocated an entirely different meaning, which will be discussed in the second half of this chapter. Meanwhile it may be defined as:

Performance: The manner or quality of functioning.

Lifestyle: A set of attitudes, habits and possessions regarded as typical of…an individual.

PHYSIOLOGICAL FACTORS

Sleep: *A state of rest during which the eyes are closed, the muscles and nerves are relaxed, and the mind is unconscious*

Elite sprinting, like every other sport, is a balance between catabolic and anabolic activity. Catabolic activity is the exercise that an athlete takes in training, which breaks down muscle tissue. Anabolic activity is the rebuilding of muscle tissue that occurs spontaneously when the athlete is sleeping and resting at home after training. An athlete usually requires at least eight hours of uninterrupted sleep each and every night to unwind and rebuild. Teenage athletes may need as many as ten hours of uninterrupted sleep each night.

Rest: *A relaxation from exertion or labour*

As well as sleep, we all need rest. Rest allows an athlete to unwind, permits further recovery, and allows a break from the mental pressures of training and competition. Rest may be active, like basketball, yoga or pilates, or sedentary or non-active, such as reading, watching television or playing video games whilst sitting or lying down. Either way, it is important that an athlete finds time to relax and 'switch off'. This gives the mind and body time to relax, helping them to be prepared and focused when competing or training.

Most emerging athletes have to combine their sport with education or a job in order to fund their present and future financial security. This might have a significant impact on the amount of leisure time available, and it is common for an athlete to have to 'juggle' his commitments in order to fit everything into his daily life.

Diet and nutrition: *The science of eating the most appropriate food to fuel an individual's lifestyle and training*

Calculating the right food to eat is covered elsewhere in this book. Here we are looking at the athlete implementing the diet by being in the right place at the right time to eat the meals that have been prepared, by allowing time for digestion, and by eating the prescribed snacks before and after training.

Smoking: *To draw the smoke of burning tobacco into the mouth and exhale it again*

Most people start smoking in order to lose weight, as a result of peer pressure, or to appear 'cool'. As athletes train hard they tend not to have weight issues; moreover as athletes they tend to be leaders and to dictate fashions rather than follow them, so few athletes smoke. Today, most people are aware of the dangers of smoking, not the least of which is lung cancer. The UK government spends nearly £23 million on attempting to stop people smoking, reflecting the costs of smoking on the National Health Service (NHS).

Alcohol: *A colourless, flammable liquid present in intoxicating drinks*

Athletes are frequently under time pressure, with training, competition and lifestyle commitments of the type discussed in this chapter. Success in competition, particularly in team sports, is frequently celebrated by binge drinking, and this is not diminished when athletes have to travel to away competitions and their only alternative is staying in their hotel to watch television. Marketing companies advertise their products as the best way to celebrate success.

Unfortunately, drinking to excess presents both short- and long-term problems. It can lead to unruly and inappropriate behaviour, with crimes sometimes committed when the person is drunk. In the long term, excessive alcohol use results in liver damage and can be fatal.

Drugs: *Substances used in the treatment, prevention or diagnosis of disease*

There are two main drugs of interest when discussing sport:

Recreational drugs: *Drugs taken for social or recreational purposes, which generally alter the mind and body. Examples include alcohol, tobacco, cannabis, cocaine and heroin*

Performance-enhancing drugs: *Drugs used by athletes to improve performance. They are strictly forbidden in sport. Examples include anabolic steroids, amphetamines and other stimulants and diuretics. Athletes may be tempted to use performance-enhancing drugs in order to achieve success. This subject is covered in another chapter*

Common recreational drugs such as marijuana, ecstasy, cocaine and heroin can be extremely dangerous and can have serious performance consequences for an athlete. Not only will performance be affected in the short term, with success unlikely, but the risk of long-term damage to health is considerable.

All athletes should avoid such drugs as there is no benefit to their use. Most recreational drugs are included in the WADA List of Prohibited Substances, so that all doping samples are also tested for recreational drugs. Athletes found positive are likely to be banned from their sport for a period of two or more years, with the possibility of a life ban for repeated offences, as well as the risk of a police prosecution and possible imprisonment. When Dwain Chambers was found to have taken a banned substance, he was banned for two years and received a lifetime ban from the Olympic Games. He was also required to return over £100,000 of prize money that he had won between the positive test and his suspension.

PSYCHOLOGICAL FACTORS

Young athletes end their junior careers and start to join senior teams and compete in senior competitions at around the age of eighteen years. This is around the age that they leave school, either to go to university or take employment. This frequently requires them to leave the family home and set up a home of their own, and to take responsibility for budgeting their own finances. They also have to find new friends near their new homes and a new boy or girl friend. All this can be very stressful and distracting from training and competition.

Independence

Living away from home: As well as leaving home to go to university or to take employment, many young athletes have to leave home in order to train and compete at the highest level. Being away from friends and family can be daunting for a young athlete, and they must be able to cope with these pressures.

Employment: Athletes have regular training and competition commitments, and require flexibility from an employer. In return, the employer who hires an athlete benefits from gaining a fit, dynamic personality, frequently popular in the local community.

Finance

Spending: Athletes are likely to combine their sport with a job in order to reach their targets. Many sports are expensive, with the costs of equipment, travel and accommodation having to be met by the athlete. Lottery funding might be available to cover the essential support services, such as coaching, training camps, competition and sport science. UK Sport also offers money to help with the essential personal living and sporting costs incurred while training and competing as an elite athlete. This is called an 'Athlete's Personal Award' (APA).

Saving: An athlete's career can be relatively short, with second careers often undertaken at the end of a competitive career. It is essential that an athlete saves some of their income so that they have a source of money in the future. Savings accounts vary greatly, with some allowing tax-free investment, while others offer immediate access to money. Either way, it is vital to have savings that you can fall back on. Savings accounts can be set up and managed online, saving a great deal of time.

Investment: Investments are forms of saving designed for longer periods of time. Money is invested in the hope of making a profit on it. Investments can come in many forms, such as buying shares in a company, or buying a property.

Tax: Paying tax can be stressful. A knowledge of what is required and how to do it is important. If you are on a fixed salary, tax should be deducted automatically before you receive your money. Any additional private work or self-employment involves declaring your income to HM Revenue and Customs. An athlete in receipt of an APA (Athlete's Personal Award) does not have to pay tax. However, if the government feels that you are a professional athlete, making a profit from sport, you will be taxed. If your sole income from sport activities is your APA, you will not be considered to be a professional athlete, so your APA is not taxable. If however, you have another source of income, you might be liable for tax. This is especially important if you receive money through sponsorship, in which case you might be taxed on your entire income.

Other financial issues requiring to be addressed are insurance and sponsorship.

Behaviour

An athlete who is regularly in the media spotlight needs to consider their role as an ambassador for their sport, as many young people will aspire to emulate them. If media pictures show the athlete smoking or behaving in an unacceptable or anti-social way, there is a possibility that children will copy that behaviour. Even amateur athletes should consider their behaviour during sporting competition and training, as well as away from the sports ground. Unruly behaviour will have a negative effect on their own image and that of their sport.

Social Life

An athlete will have many pressures that affect the amount of time they have available to spend with friends and family. However, it is important that time is spent relaxing in their company, away from the pressures of training and competition. The athlete's training programme should include time to relax and socialize.

GAMBLING

Gambling on sport is a multi-billion pound industry. Some sports, such as greyhound racing and horse racing, are dominated by gambling. The development of the internet has allowed gambling to become more accessible, and there has been a significant rise in the profile of the industry. It is now common for football teams to be sponsored by gambling companies.

Athletes are not allowed to gamble on events in which they are involved, and there are strict laws to enforce this. This is to prevent allegations of match fixing, where the result is determined not by skill, but by cheating. Cricketers and footballers have both recently been convicted of offences in relation to match-fixing scandals.

High-earning athletes often gamble on sports in order to get the same thrill that they get when they are successful in their own performance. You will probably be familiar with a number of media cases where famous athletes have gambled large amounts of money at sporting events. Attention is often focused on the amount they bet and the amount of money lost.

Because betting is risky, it is easy to lose money quickly. Proper financial investment is a much better option.

Stress and Anxiety

Stress: Stress is a mental or physical response to a situation that an athlete feels they cannot cope with. Symptoms will be characterized by increased heart rate, a rise in blood pressure, muscular tension, irritability and depression.

Anxiety: Anxiety is a negative form of stress that is characterized by long-term feelings of low confidence and poor concentration. Common symptoms will be a fear of failure and low self-esteem. Anxiety is likely to reduce the athlete's level of performance.

THE ENGLISH INSTITUTE OF SPORT (EIS) CONCEPT OF PERFORMANCE LIFESTYLE

The English Institute of Sport (EIS) was formed by Sport England in 2002, with plans to invest an annual budget of £120 million to assist elite athletes to be as good as they could be. This substantial budget allowed the EIS to define a new area, which it called 'performance lifestyle', where it could do this. Their definition of performance lifestyle is as follows:

Performance lifestyle is a personalized support service specifically designed to help each athlete create the unique environment necessary for their success. For elite athletes to maintain a performance lifestyle they must fit many aspects of their life alongside their intensive training programme. Trained and accredited athlete advisers at the EIS aim to provide support to athletes by giving them the necessary skills to cope with the special demands of being an elite performer and to better prepare them for their life after sport.

The approach is to work closely with coaches and support specialists as part of an integrated team to minimize potential concerns, conflicts and distractions, all of which can be detrimental to performance, and at worst, may end a sport career prematurely. Performance lifestyle advisers can support athletes with time management, budgeting and finance, dealing with the media, sponsorship and negotiation/conflict management. Advice is also available for athletes on finding suitable jobs.

This definition means that the EIS does not get involved in the work of the athlete's coaches or with any potential disciplinary action of the athlete in connection with cigarettes, alcohol or drugs, but rather focuses on giving legal, financial and management advice to athletes on subjects such as:

- time management
- budgeting and finance
- dealing with the media
- sponsorship and promotion activities
- negotiation/conflict management

Manchester United Football Club has run a Player Support Office for many years. The office is open twenty-four hours a day, seven days a week and fifty-two weeks a year, to support players with all types of problems, from delivering and collecting dry cleaning to finding child minders for players' children and even arranging legal representation at a police station if a player is arrested. Having players worth £80 million on their payroll, such as Cristiano Ronaldo before his move to Real Madrid, they clearly want to protect their investments.

The EIS service is clearly very basic when

compared to the Manchester United office, but the staffing and resources available at the 'World's Wealthiest Football Club' exceed anything available to the English Institute of Sport. It is also a great advantage that all the footballers live relatively close to the club, rather than being spread all over the United Kingdom of Great Britain and Northern Ireland, and even, on occasion, in other countries for work, education or training camps. If the EIS is able to assist just one or two athletes to resolve problems and to win medals, then it will justify its cost to the tax payers.

REFERENCES

A & C Black Publishers Ltd *Dictionary of Sport and Exercise Science*, 2006 (London: A & C Black Publishers Ltd ISBN-13:978-0713677850)

Abbiss, C. R. and Laursen, P. B. 'Describing and understanding pacing strategies during athletic competition' 2008, *Sports Medicine*, 38(3), 239–252

Abraham, A., and Collins, D. 'Taking the next step: Ways forward for coaching science' 2011, *Quest*, 63(4), 366–384

Ackerman, P. L. 'Predicting individual differences in complex skill acquisition: dynamics of ability determinants' 1992, *Journal of Applied Psychology*, 77(5), 598

Aggen, P. D. and Reuteman, P. 'Conservative rehabilitation of sciatic nerve injury following hamstring tear' 2010, North American journal of sports physical therapy: *NAJSPT*, 5(3), 143

Alexandrov, I. and Lucht, P. 'Physics of sprinting' 1981, *American Journal of Physics*, 49(3), 254–257

Alfredson, H. Ultrasound and Doppler-guided minisurgery to treat midportion Achilles tendinosis: results of a large material and a randomized study comparing two scraping techniques 2011, *British Journal of Sports Medicine* 45(5), 407–410. doi: 10.1136/bjsm.2010.081216

Alfredson, H. and Lorentzon, R. 'Chronic achilles tendinosis: recommendations for treatment and prevention 2000, *Sports Medicine*, 29(2), 135–146

Atwater, A. E. 'Kinematic analyses of sprinting' 1982, *Track and Field Quarterly Review*, 82(2), 12–16

Baechle, T. R. and Earle, R. *Weight Training (Steps to Success)* 2006 (Champaign, IL: Human Kinetics Publishers. ISBN-13:978-0736055338)

Baker, J. and Cobley, S. 'Outliers, talent codes and myths', in Farrow, D., Baker, J. and MacMahon, C. (eds) 'Developing Sport Expertise: Researchers and coaches put theory into practice' 2013 (Routledge, pp 13–30)

Barton, M. C. J., Munteanu, S. E., Menz, H. B. and Crossley, K. M. 'The efficacy of foot orthoses in the treatment of individuals with patellofemoral pain syndrome' 2010, *Sports Medicine*, 40(5), 377–395

Bassons, C., Hopquin, B. and Cossins, P. *A Clean Break: My Story* 2014 (London: Bloomsbury Sport ISBN-13:978-1472910356)

Baumann, W. 'Kinematic and dynamic characteristics of the sprint start' 1976, *Biomechanics V* Vol. B, 194–199

Baumeister, R. F. 'Choking under pressure: self-consciousness and paradoxical effects of incentives on skilful performance' 1984, *Journal of Personality and Social Psychology*, 46(3), 610–620

Bergh, U., Thorstensson, A., Sjödin, B. E. R. T. I. L., Hulten, B. O. D. I. L., Piehl, K. A. R. I. N. and Karlsson, J. 'Maximal oxygen uptake and muscle fiber types in trained and untrained humans' 1977, *Medicine and Science in Sports*, 10 (3), 151–154

Bloom, B. S. 'Generalizations about talent development. Developing talent in young people' 1985, 507–549

Bloomer, R. J., Larson, D. E., Fisher-Wellman, K. H., Galpin, A. J. and Schilling, B. K. 'Effect of eicosapentaenoic and docosahexaenoic acid on resting and exercise-induced inflammatory and oxidative stress biomarkers: a randomized, placebo-controlled, cross-over study' 2009, *Lipids in Health and Disease* 8(1), 36

Borzov, V. P. 1978. 'Contest lasts seconds' (Kyiv: Veselka)

Bruggeman, G. P., Koszewski, D., and Muller, H. 'Biomechanical research project: Athens 1997 – Final Report, International Athletic Federation, Oxford, UK' 1999, *Meyer & Meyer Sport*

Burkett, B. *Sport Mechanics for Coaches* (3rd edition) 2010 (Champaign, IL: Human Kinetics Publishers ASIN: B00E2800)

Burkett, B. 'Technology in Paralympic sport: performance enhancement or essential for performance?' 2010, *British Journal of Sports Medicine*, 44(3), 215–220

Cacchio, A., Rompe, J. D., Furia, J. P., Susi, P., Santilli, V., and De Paulis, F. 'Shockwave therapy for the treatment of chronic proximal hamstring tendinopathy in professional athletes' 2011, *The American Journal of Sports Medicine*, 39(1), 146–153, doi: 10.1177/0363546510379324

Cameron, M. L., Adams, R. D., Maher, C. G. and Misson, D. 'Effect of the HamSprint Drills training programme on lower limb neuromuscular control in Australian football players' 2009, *Journal of Science and Medicine in Sport*, 12(1), 24–30. doi: 10.1016/j.jsams.2007.09.003

Carr, A. J., Hopkins, W. G. and Gore, C. J. 'Effects of acute alkalosis and acidosis on performance' 2011, *Sports Medicine*, 41(10), 801–814

Carrillon, Y. and Cohen, M. 'Imaging findings of muscle traumas in sports medicine' 2007, Journal de Radiologie, 88 (1 Pt 2), 129–142

Casey, A., and Greenhaff, P. L. 'Does dietary creatine supplementation play a role in skeletal muscle metabolism and performance?' 2000, *The American Journal of Clinical Nutrition*, 72(2), 607s–617s

Chen, Z. P., Stephens, T. J., Murthy, S., Canny, B. J., Hargreaves, M., Witters, L. A. and McConell, G. K. 'Effect of exercise intensity on skeletal muscle AMPK signaling in humans' 2003, *Diabetes*, 52(9), 2,205–2,212

Clanton, T. O. and Coupe, K. J. 'Hamstring strains in athletes: diagnosis and treatment' 1998, *Journal of the American Academy of Orthopaedic Surgeons*, 6(4), 237–248

Clarke, S. F., Murphy, E. F., O'Sullivan, O., Lucey, A. J., Humphreys, M., Hogan, A., ... and Cotter, P. D. 'Exercise and associated dietary extremes impact on gut microbial diversity' 2014, Gut, gutjnl-2013

Coffey, V. G., Moore, D. R., Burd, N. A., Rerecich, T., Stellingwerff, T., Garnham, A. P., ... and Hawley, J. A. 'Nutrient provision increases signalling and protein synthesis in human skeletal muscle after repeated sprints' 2011, *European Journal of Applied Physiology*, 111(7), 1,473–1,483

Čoh, M., Jošt, B., Škof, B., Tomažin, K., and Dolenec, A. 'Kinematic and kinetic parameters of the sprint start and start acceleration model of top sprinters' 1998, *Gymnica*, 28, 33–42

Čoh, M., Peharec, S. and Bacic, P. 'The sprint start: Biomechanical analysis of kinematic, dynamic and electromyographic parameters' 2007, *New Studies in Athletics*, 22(3), 29

Čoh, M., Tomažin, K. and Štuhec, S. 'The biomechanical model of the sprint start and block acceleration' 2006, Facta universitatis-series: *Physical Education and Sport*, 4(2), 103–114

Cohn, P. J. 'Preperformance Routines in Sport: Theoretical Support and Practical Applications' 1990, *Sport Psychologist*, 4(3) 301–312

Collet, C. 'Strategic aspects of reaction time in world-class sprinters' 1999, *Perceptual and Motor Skills*, 88(1), 65–75

Collins, D., and Cruickshank, A. 'The P7 approach to the Olympic challenge: Getting things as right as possible, for as many as possible, as often as possible' 2014, *International Journal of Sport and Exercise Psychology*. Manuscript under review

Collins, D. and MacNamara, Á. 'The rocky road to the top' 2012, *Sports Medicine*, 42(11), 907–914

Conte, V. *Balco: The Straight Dope on Steroids* 2008 (New York: Skyhorse Publishing ISBN-13:978-1602392953)

Cooke, N. *The Breakaway* 2014 (London: Simon & Schuster UK ASIN:B00DJWA0OW)

Cooper, C. *Run, Swim, Throw, Cheat: The science behind drugs in sport* 2013 (Oxford: Oxford University Press ISBN-13:978-0199678785)

Copland, S. T., Tipton, J. S. and Fields, K. B. 'Evidence-based treatment of hamstring tears' 2009, current sports medicine reports, 8(6), 308–314, doi: 10.1249/JSR.0b013e3181c1d6e1

Coppenolle, H., Delecluse, C., Goris, M., Diels, R. and Kraayenhof, H. 'An evaluation of the starting action of world class female sprinters' 1990, *Track Technique*, 90, 3,581–3,582

Costill, D. L., Flynn, M. G., Kirwan, J. P., Houmard, J. A., Mitchell, J. B., Thomas, R. and Park, S. H. 'Effects of repeated days of intensified training on muscle glycogen and swimming performance' 1988, *Medicine and Science in Sports and Exercise*, 20(3), 249–254

Cousins, S. and Dyson, R. 'Forces at the front and rear blocks during the sprint start' 2008, March. In ISBS-Conference Proceedings Archive (Vol. 1, No. 1)

Creer, A., Gallagher, P., Slivka, D., Jemiolo, B., Fink, W. and Trappe, S. 'Influence of muscle glycogen availability on ERK1/2 and Akt signaling after resistance exercise in human skeletal muscle' 2005, *Journal of Applied Physiology*, 99(3), 950–956

Cribb, P. J. and Hayes, A. 'Effects of Supplement-Timing and Resistance Exercise on Skeletal Muscle Hypertrophy' 2006, *Medicine & Science in Sports & Exercise*, 38(11), 1,918–1,925

Cribb, P. J., Williams, A. D. and Hayes, A. 'A creatine-protein-carbohydrate supplement enhances responses to resistance training' 2007, *Medicine and Science in Sport and Exercise*, 39(11), 1,960–1,968

Dallinga, J. M., Benjaminse, A and Lemmink, K. A. 'Which Screening Tools Can Predict Injury to the

Lower Extremities in Team Sports?' 2012, *Sports Medicine*, 42(9), 791-815. doi: 10.2165/11632730-000000000-00000

Daneshjoo, A., Rahnama, N., Mokhtar, A. H. and Yusof, A. 'Bilateral and unilateral asymmetries of isokinetic strength and flexibility in male young professional soccer players' 2013, *Journal of Human Kinetics*, 36(1), 45–53. doi: 10.2478/hukin-2013-0005

Davis, J. K. and Green, J. M. 'Caffeine and anaerobic performance' 2009, *Sports Medicine*, 39(10), 813–832

de Koning, J. J., Bobbert, M. F. and Foster, C. 'Determination of optimal pacing strategy in track cycling with an energy flow model' 1999, *Journal of Science and Medicine in Sport*, 2(3), 266–277

Delavier, F. *Women's Strength Training Anatomy* 2002 (Champaign, IL: Human Kinetics Europe Ltd, ISBN-13:978-0736048132)

Delavier, F. *Strength Training Anatomy* 2010 (Champaign, IL: Human Kinetics Publishers ISBN-13:978-0736092265)

Dick, F. W. *Sprints and Relays* 1987 (British Amateur Athletic Board ISBN-13: 978-0851340821)

Dick, F. W. *Sports Training Principles* (4th edition) 2002 (London: A & C Black Publishers Ltd ISBN-13:978-0713658651)

Dierks, T. A., Manal, K. T., Hamill, J. and Davis, I. 'Lower extremity kinematics in runners with patellofemoral pain during a prolonged run' 2011, *Medicine and Science in Sports and Exercise*, 43(4), 693–700

Dorling Kindersley *Strength Training* 2009 (London: Dorling Kindersley ISBN-13:978-1405344371)

Doscher, W. *The Art of Sprinting: Techniques for Speed and Performance* 2009 (McFarland & Co Inc. ISBN-13: 978-0786443147)

Dragoo, J. L., Johnson, C. and McConnell, J. 'Evaluation and treatment of disorders of the infrapatellar fat pad' 2012, *Sports Medicine*, 42(1), 51–67. doi: 10.2165/11595680-000000000-00000.

Drechsler, A. J. *The Weightlifting Encyclopedia: A Guide to World Class Performance* 1998 (USA: A is A Communications ISBN-13:978-0965917926)

Dreyer, H. C., Drummond, M. J., Pennings, B., Fujita, S., Glynn, E. L., Chinkes, D. L., and Rasmussen, B. B. 'Leucine-enriched essential amino acid and carbohydrate ingestion following resistance exercise enhances mTOR signaling and protein synthesis in human muscle' 2008, *American Journal of Physiology-Endocrinology And Metabolism*, 294(2), E392–E400

Drummond, M. J. and Rasmussen, B. B. 'Leucine-enriched nutrients and the regulation of mammalian target of rapamycin signalling and human skeletal muscle protein synthesis 2008, *Current Opinion in Clinical Nutrition & Metabolic Care*, 11(3), 222–226

Duckworth, A. L., Peterson, C., Matthews, M. D., & Kelly, D. R. 'Grit: perseverance and passion for long-term goals' 2007, *Journal of Personality and Social Psychology*, 92(6), 1,087–1,101

Edwards, J. *Research in Sprinting ~ What Science Says About Speed* 2012 (New American Press ASIN: B008BO0TX0)

Edwards, W. *An introduction to motor learning and motor control* 2011 (Wadsworth)

Elfrink, T. *Blood Sport: Alex Rodriguez, Biogenesis, and the Quest to End Baseball's Steroid Era* 2014 (London: Dutton Books ISBN-13:978-0525954637)

Ellis, R., Hing, W. and Reid, D. 'Iliotibial band friction syndrome—a systematic review' 2007, *Manual Therapy*, 12(3), 200–208. doi: 10.1016/j.math.2006.08.004

Epstein, D. *The Sports Gene: Inside the Science of Extraordinary Athletic Performance* 2014 (N.Y.: Current, ASIN:B00KEM94MO)

Ericsson, K. A., Krampe, R. T. and Tesch-Römer, C. 'The role of deliberate practice in the acquisition of expert performance' 1993, *Psychological Review*, 100(3), 363

Fahlström, M., Jonsson, P., Lorentzon, R. and Alfredson, H. 'Chronic Achilles tendon pain treated with eccentric calf-muscle training' 2003, *Knee Surgery, Sports Traumatology, Arthroscopy*, 11(5), 327–333, doi: 10.1007/s00167-003-0418-z

Filby, W. C., Maynard, I. W. and Graydon, J. K. 'The effect of multiple-goal strategies on performance outcomes in training and competition' 1999, *Journal of Applied Sport Psychology*, 11(2), 230–246

Fleischman, E. A., Quaintance, M. K. and Broedling, L. A. *Taxonomies of Human Performance: The Description of Human Tasks* 1984 (Orlando, FL: Academic Press Inc. ISBN-13: 978-0122604508)

Fleishman, E. A. 'On the relation between abilities, learning, and human performance' 1972, *American Psychologist*, 27(11), 1,017

Fortier, S., Basset, F. A., Mbourou, G. A., Favérial, J. and Teasdale, N. 'Starting block performance in sprinters: A statistical method for identifying discriminative parameters of the performance and an analysis of the effect of providing feedback over a 6-week period' 2005, *Journal of Sports Science and Medicine*, 4(2), 134

Fujita, S., Dreyer, H. C., Drummond, M. J., Glynn, E. L., Cadenas, J. G., Yoshizawa, F., and Rasmussen, B. B. 'Nutrient signalling in the regulation of human muscle protein synthesis' 2007, *The Journal of Physiology*, 582(2), 813–823

Gibala, M. J., McGee, S. L., Garnham, A. P., Howlett, K. F., Snow, R. J., and Hargreaves, M. 'Brief intense interval exercise activates AMPK and p38

MAPK signaling and increases the expression of PGC-1α in human skeletal muscle' 2009, *Journal of Applied Physiology*, 106(3), 929–934

Gittoes, M. J. and Wilson, C. 'Intralimb joint coordination patterns of the lower extremity in maximal velocity phase sprint running' 2010, *Journal of Applied Biomechanics*, 2, 188–195

Goldstein, E. R., Ziegenfuss, T., Kalman, D., Kreider, R., Campbell, B., Wilborn, C., and Antonio, J. 'International society of sports nutrition position stand: caffeine and performance' 2010, *J Int Soc Sports Nutr*, 7(1), 5

Guissard, N., Duchateau, J. and Hainaut, K. 'EMG and mechanical changes during sprint starts at different front block obliquities' 1992, *Medicine and Science in Sports and Exercise*, 24(11), 1,257–1,263

Guissard, N., Duchateau, J. 'Electromyography of the sprint start' 1990, *J. Of Human Movement Studies*, 18, 97–106

Hackney, A. C., Pearman, S. N. and Novack, J. M. 'Physiological profiles of overstrained and stale athletes, A review' 1990, *Applied Sport Psychology*, 2, 21–30

Hafez, A. M. A., Roberts, E. M. and Seireg, A. A. 'Force and velocity during front foot contact in the sprint start' 1985, *International Series On Biomechanics*, 5, 350–355

Hamill, J., van Emmerik, R. E., Heiderscheit, B. C. and Li, L. 'A dynamical systems approach to lower extremity running injuries' 1999, *Clinical Biomechanics*, 14(5), 297–308

Hanin, Y. L. 'Emotions in sport: Current issues and perspectives' 2007, *Handbook of Sport Psychology*, 3, 31–58

Hardy, L., Jones, J. G., and Gould, D. 'Understanding psychological preparation for sport: Theory and practice of elite performers' 1996, John Wiley & Sons Inc. Chichester

Hardy, L., Mullen, R., and Jones, G. 'Knowledge and conscious control of motor actions under stress' 1996, *British Journal of Psychology*, 87(4), 621–636

Harland, M. J. and Steele, J. R. 'Biomechanics of the sprint start' 1997, *Sports Medicine*, 23(1), 11–20

Hartman, J. W., Moore, D. R. and Phillips, S. M. 'Resistance training reduces whole-body protein turnover and improves net protein retention in untrained young males' 2006, *Applied Physiology, Nutrition, and Metabolism*, 31(5), 557–564

Hay, J. G. *The Biomechanics of Sports Techniques* (4th edition), 1993 (Benjamin Cummings ISBN-13: 978-0130845344)

Hettinga, F. J., De Koning, J. J., Broersen, F. T., Van Geffen, P. and Foster, C. 'Pacing strategy and the occurrence of fatigue in 4000m cycling time trials' 2006, *Medicine and Science in Sports and Exercise*, 38(8), 1484

Hill, C. A., Harris, R. C., Kim, H. J., Harris, B. D., Sale, C., Boobis, L. H., and Wise, J. A. 'Influence of β-alanine supplementation on skeletal muscle carnosine concentrations and high intensity cycling capacity' 2007, *Amino acids*, 32(2), 225–233

Hinrichs, R. N., Cavanagh, P. R. and Williams, K. R. 'Upper Extremity Function in Running. I: Center of Mass and Propulsion Considerations' 1987, *International Journal of Sport Biomechanics*, 3(3)

Hodges, N. and Williams, M. A. *Skill Acquisition in Sport: Research, Theory and Practice*, 2nd edition, 2012 (London: Routledge. ISBN-13: 978-0415607865)

Holmes, P. S., and Collins, D. J. 'The PETTLEP approach to motor imagery: A functional equivalence model for sport psychologists' 2001, *Journal of Applied Sport Psychology*, 13(1), 60–83

Hoskins, W. and Pollard, H. 'Hamstring injury management – Part 2: Treatment' 2005a, *Manual Therapy*, 10(3), 180–190. doi: 10.1016/j.math.2005.05.001

Hoskins, W. and Pollard, H. 'The management of hamstring injury – Part 1: Issues in diagnosis' 2005b, *Manual Therapy*, 10(2), 96–107. doi: 10.1016/ j.math.2005.03.006

Hoster, M. and May, E. 'Notes on the biomechanics of the sprint start' 1979, *Athletics Coach*, 13(2), 2–7

Hughes, M. and Franks, I. *The Essentials of Performance Analysis: An Introduction* 2007 (London: Routledge ISBN-13:978-0415423809)

Husbands, C. *Sprinting: Training, Techniques and Improving Performance* 2013 (Crowood Press ISBN-13: 978-1847975492)

Johnson, C., Paish, W. and Dick, F. *Strength Training for Athletics* 1978, instructional book: British Amateur Athletic Board ASIN: B001DI8LIQ

Jones, A. M. 'Running economy is negatively related to sit-and-reach test performance in international-standard distance runners' 2002 *International Journal of Sports Medicine*, 23(01), 40–43

Jones, G. 'The role of performance profiling in cognitive behavioural interventions in sport' 1993, *Sport Psychologist*, 7, 160–172

Jones, R., Bezodis, I. and Thompson, A. 'Coaching sprinting: expert coaches' perception of race phases and technical constructs' 2009, *International Journal of Sports Science and Coaching*, 4(3), 385–396

Keller, J. B. 'A theory of competitive running' 1973, *Physics Today*, 43

Keller, J. B. 'Optimal velocity in a race' 1974, *American Mathematical Monthly*, 474–480

Kellmann, M. *Enhancing Recovery: Preventing Under Performance in Athletics* 2002 (Champaign, IL: Human Kinetics Publishers ISBN-13:978-0736034005)

Kilcoyne, K. G., Dickens, J. F., Keblish, D., Rue, J. P. and Chronister, R. 'Outcome of Grade I and II Hamstring Injuries in Intercollegiate Athletes: A Novel Rehabilitation Protocol' 2011, *Sports Health: A Multidisciplinary Approach*, 3(6), 528–533. doi: 10.1177/1941738111422044

Kimball, S. R. and Jefferson, L. S. 'Signaling pathways and molecular mechanisms through which branched-chain amino acids mediate translational control of protein synthesis' 2006, *The Journal of Nutrition*, 136(1), 227S–231S

Kimball, S. R. and Jefferson, L. S. 'Control of translation initiation through integration of signals generated by hormones, nutrients, and exercise' 2010, *Journal of Biological Chemistry*, 285(38), 29,027–29,032

Korchemny, R. 'A new concept of sprint start and acceleration training' 1992, *New Studies in Athletics*, 7(4), 65–72

Korhonen, M. T., Mero, A. and Suominen, H. 'Age-related differences in 100m sprint performance in male and female master runners' 2003, *Medicine and Science in Sports and Exercise*, 35(8), 1,419–1,428

Kraemer, W. J. and Fleck, S. J. *Designing Resistance Training Programs* (3rd edition) 2003 (Champaign, IL: Human Kinetics Publishers ISBN-13:978-0736042574)

Kraemer, W. J. and Fleck, S. J. *Strength Training for Young Athletes* 2004 (Champaign, IL: Human Kinetics Publishers. ISBN-13:978-0736051033)

Krustrup, P., Mohr, M., Steensberg, A., Bencke, J., Kjær, M. and Bangsbo, J. 'Muscle and blood metabolites during a soccer game: implications for sprint performance' 2006, *Medicine and Science in Sports and Exercise*, 38(6), 1,165–1,174

Laird, P. and Waters, L. 'Eyewitness recollection of sport coaches' 2008, *International Journal of Performance Analysis in Sport*, 8(1), 76–84

Lam, W. K., Maxwell, J. P., and Masters, R. 'Analogy learning and the performance of motor skills under pressure' 2009, *Journal of Sport and Exercise Psychology*, 31(3), 337–357

Lambert, C. P. and Flynn, M. G. 'Fatigue during high-intensity intermittent exercise' 2002, *Sports Medicine*, 32(8), 511–522

Lee, E. S. and Whitfield, J. *Fundamentals of Sprinting* 2010 (Xlibris Corporation ISBN-13: 978-1441599001)

Linthorne, N. 'Wind assistance in the 100m sprint' 1994, *Track Technique*, 127, 4049–4051

Locke, E. A. 'Motivation through conscious goal setting' 1996, *Applied and Preventive Psychology*, 5(2), 117–124

Locke, E. A. and Latham, G. P. 'The application of goal setting to sports' 1985, *Journal of Sport Psychology*, 7(3), 205–222

Locke, E. A. and Latham, G. P. *Goal Setting: A Motivational Technique that Works* 1984 (Englewood Cliffs, NJ: Prentice Hall: ISBN-13:978-0133574678)

Lombardo, M. P. and Deaner, R. O. 'You Can't Teach Speed: Sprinters Falsify the Deliberate Practice Model of Expertise' 2013 (available at SSRN 2277977)

Longo, U. G., Ronga, M. and Maffulli, N. 'Achilles tendinopathy' 2009, *Sports medicine and arthroscopy review*, 17(2), 112–126. doi: 10.1097/JSA.0b013e3181a3d625

Macnamara, Á., and Collins, D. 'Development and initial validation of the Psychological Characteristics of Developing Excellence Questionnaire' 2011, *Journal of Sports Sciences*, 29(12), 1,273–1,286

MacNamara, Á., Button, A. and Collins, D. 'The Role of Psychological Characteristics in Facilitating the Pathway to Elite Performance: Part 1: Identifying Mental Skills and Behaviors' 2010a, *The Sport Psychologist*, 24(1), 52–73

MacNamara, Á., Button, A. and Collins, D. 'The Role of Psychological Characteristics in Facilitating the Pathway to Elite Performance: Part 2: Examining Environmental and Stage-Related Differences in Skills and Behaviors' 2010b, *The Sport Psychologist*, 24(1), 74–96

MacPherson, A. C., Collins, D. and Morriss, C. 'Is what you think what you get? Optimizing mental focus for technical performance' 2008, *The Sport Psychologist*, 22(3), 288–303

MacPherson, A. C., Collins, D. and Obhi, S. S. 'The importance of temporal structure and rhythm for the optimum performance of motor skills: a new focus for practitioners of sport psychology' 2009, *Journal of Applied Sport Psychology*, 21(S1), S48–S61

Macur, J. *Cycle of Lies: The Fall of Lance Armstrong* 2014 (London: Williams Collins ISBN-13: 978-0007520633)

Malina, R. M., Bouchard, C. and Bar-Or, O. *Growth, Maturation and Physical Activity* (2nd edition) 2004 (Champaign, IL: Human Kinetics Publishers ISBN-13: 978-0880118828)

Mann, R. *The Mechanics of Sprinting and Hurdling* 2011 (CreateSpace Independent Publishing Platform ISBN-13: 978-1461136316)

Mann, R. V. 'A kinetic analysis of sprinting' 1980 *Medicine and Science in Sports and Exercise*, 13(5), 325–328

Mann, R., Kotmel, J., Herman, J., Johnson, B. and Schultz, C. 'Kinematic trends in elite sprinters' 2008, March. In ISBS-Conference Proceedings Archive (Vol. 1, No. 1)

Manore, M. M., Barr, S. I. and Butterfield, G. A. 'Nutrition and athletic performance. A joint position statement of the American Dietetic Association, the Dietitians of Canada, and the American College of Sports Medicine' 2000 *Med. Sci. Sports Exerc*, 32, 2,130–2,145

Maquirriain, J. 'Surgical treatment of chronic Achilles tendinopathy: long-term results of the endoscopic technique' 2013 *The Journal of Foot and Ankle Surgery*, 52(4), 451–455. doi: 10.1053/j.jfas.2013.03.031

Marlow, B. *Sprinting and Relay Racing* 1966 (British Amateur Athletic Board. ASIN: B0014MB0JI)

Marlow, B. *Sprinting and Relay Racing: Instruction Book* 1977 (British Amateur Athletic Board ASIN: B001OJTOTE)

Martindale, A. and Collins, D. 'Professional judgment and decision making: the role of intention for impact' 2005 *Sport Psychologist* 19(3), 303–317

Martindale, A. and Collins, D. 'A professional judgment and decision making case study: Reflection-in-action research' 2012 *The Sport Psychologist*, 26, 500–518

Masters, R. S. 'Knowledge, knerves and knowhow: the role of explicit versus implicit knowledge in the breakdown of a complex motor skill under pressure' 1992 *British journal of psychology*, 83(3), 343–358

McArdle, W. D., Katch, F. I. and Katch, V. L. *Exercise Physiology: Energy, Nutrition and Human Performance* 1996 (Lippincott Williams and Wilkins ISBN-13:978-0683057317)

McConnell, J. 'The physical therapist's approach to patellofemoral disorders' 2002 *Clinics in Sports Medicine*, 21(3), 363–387

McNab, T. *Modern Schools Athletics* 1971 (Hodder Arnold H&S ISBN-13: 978-0340152607)

McNab, T. *Complete Book of Athletics* 1980 (Littlehampton: Littlehampton Book Services Ltd ISBN-13: 978-0706359275)

McNab, T. *Successful Track Athletics* 1982 (Littlehampton: Littlehampton Book Services Ltd ISBN-13: 978-0850974171)

McNab, T. and Gifford, D. *Speed: Gain Athletic Speed for Improved Track and Field Performance* 1989 (Sackville Books ISBN-13: 978-0948615238)

Mendiguchia, J., Alentorn-Geli, E., Idoate, F. and Myer, G. D. 'Rectus femoris muscle injuries in football: a clinically relevant review of mechanisms of injury, risk factors and preventive strategies' 2012 *British Journal of Sports Medicine* 47(6), 359–366. doi: 10.1136/bjsports-2012-091250.

Mero, A. 'Force-time characteristics and running velocity of male sprinters during the acceleration phase of sprinting' 1988 *Research Quarterly for Exercise and Sport*, 59(2), 94–98

Mero, A. and Komi, P. V. 'Reaction time and electromyographic activity during a sprint start' 1990 *European Journal of Applied Physiology and Occupational Physiology* 61 (1–2), 73–80

Mero, A., Kuitunen, S., Harland, M., Kyröläinen, H. and Komi, P. V. 'Effects of muscle–tendon length on joint moment and power during sprint starts' 2006 *Journal of Sports Sciences* 24 (2), 165–173

Mero, A., Luhtanen, P. and Komi, P. V. 'A biomechanical study of the sprint start' 1983 *Scandinavian Journal of Sports Science* 5 (1), 20–28

Moore, R. *The Dirtiest Race in History: Ben Johnson, Carl Lewis and the 1988 Olympic 100m Final* 2013 (London: Wisden Sports Writing ISBN-13:978-1408158760)

Morin, J. B., Dalleau, G., Kyrolainen, H., Jeannin, T. and Belli, A. 'A simple method for measuring stiffness during running' 2005 *Journal of Applied Biomechanics* 21 (2), 167–180

Mottram, D. R. *Drugs in Sport* (5th edition) 2010 (London: Routledge ISBN-13:978-0415550871)

National Strength and Conditioning Association *Exercise Technique Manual for Resistance Training* 2008 (Champaign, IL: Human Kinetics Europe Ltd ISBN-13:978-0736071277)

Newton, H. *Explosive Lifting for Sports* 2002 (Champaign, IL: Human Kinetics Publishers ISBN-13:978-0736041720)

Noreen, E. E., Sass, M. J., Crowe, M. L., Pabon, V. A., Brandauer, J. and Averill, L. K. 'Effects of supplemental fish oil on resting metabolic rate, body composition, and salivary cortisol in healthy adults' 2010 *Journal of the International Society of Sports Nutrition* 7 (31), 10–1186

O'Donoghue, P. Time-motion analysis, in Hughes, M. and Franks, I. (2007) *The essentials of performance analysis: an introduction* 2008 (London: Routledge ISBN-13: 978-0415423809)

O'Reilly, E. *The Race to Truth: Blowing the whistle on Lance Armstrong and cycling's doping culture* 2014 (London: Bantam Press ISBN-13:978-0593074060)

OUP *Oxford Dictionary of Sports Science and Medicine* (3rd edition) 2006 (Oxford: Oxford University Press ISBN-13:978-0199210893)

Paish, W. *Introduction to Athletics* 1974 (Faber & Faber ISBN-13: 978-0571101917)

Paish, W. *Diet in Sport* 1979 (EP Publishing Ltd ISBN-13: 978-0715806586)

Paish, W. *Training for Peak Performance (Other Sports)* 1991 (A & C Black Publishers Ltd ISBN-13: 978-0713634044)

Paish, W. *Complete Manual of Sports Science: A Practical Guide to Applied Sports Science (Nutrition and Fitness)* 1998 (A & C Black Publishers Ltd ISBN-13: 978-0713648546)

Paish, W. and Duffy, T. *Athletics in Focus* 1976 (Lepus Books ISBN-13: 978-0860190103)

Palmieri-Smith, R. M., Kreinbrink, J., Ashton-Miller, J. A. and Wojtys, E. M. 'Quadriceps inhibition induced by an experimental knee joint effusion affects knee joint mechanics during a single-legged drop landing' 2007 *The American Journal of Sports Medicine* 35(8), 1,269–1,275 doi: 10.1177/0363546506296417)

Payne, A. H. and Blader, F. B. 'The mechanics of the sprint start' 1971 *Biomechanics II* 225–231

Payne, V. G., Isaacs, L. D. and Pohlman, R. *Human motor development: A lifespan approach* 2002 (pp. 365–390) (Boston: McGraw-Hill)

Peers, K. H. and Lysens, R. J. 'Patellar tendinopathy in athletes' 2005 *Sports Medicine* 35 (1), 71–87

Puranen, J. and Orava, S. 'The hamstring syndrome: A new diagnosis of gluteal sciatic pain' 1988 *The American Journal of Sports Medicine* 16 (5), 517–521

Quinn, M. D. 'External effects in the 400m hurdles race' 2010 *Journal of Applied Biomechanics* 26 (2)

Richter, E. and Ruderman, N. 'AMPK and the biochemistry of exercise: implications for human health and disease' 2009 *Biochemistry Journal* 418, 261–275

Rundqvist, H. C., Lilja, M. R., Rooyackers, O., Odrzywol, K., Murray, J. T., Esbjörnsson, M. and Jansson, E. 'Nutrient ingestion increased mTOR signaling, but not hVps34 activity in human skeletal muscle after sprint exercise' 2013 *Physiological reports* 1(5).

Rushall, B. S. and Potgieter, J. R. *The Psychology of Successful Competing in Endurance Events* 1987 (South African Association for Sport Science, Physical Education and Recreation, Pretoria)

Sale, C., Saunders, B. and Harris, R. C. 'Effect of beta-alanine supplementation on muscle carnosine concentrations and exercise performance' 2010 *Amino acids* 39 (2), 321–333

Salo, A. I., Bezodis, I. N., Batterham, A. M. and Kerwin, D. G. 'Elite sprinting: are athletes individually step-frequency or step-length reliant?' 2011 *Medicine and Science in Sports and Exercise* 43 (6), 1055–1062

Schache, A. G., Dorn, T. W., Blanch, P. D., Brown, N. A. and Pandy, M. G. 'Mechanics of the human hamstring muscles during sprinting' 2012 *Medicine and Science in Sports and Exercise* 44 (4), 647–658. doi: 10.1249/MSS.0b013e318236a3d2

Schache, A. G., Wrigley, T. V., Baker, R. and Pandy, M. G. 'Biomechanical response to hamstring muscle strain injury' 2009 *Gait and Posture* 29(2), 332–338 doi: 10.1016/ j.gaitpost.2008.10.054

Schmidt, R. and Lee, T. *Motor Control and Learning* (5th edition) 2011 (Champaign, IL: Human Kinetics Publishers ISBN-13: 978-0736079617)

Schmidt, R. and Wrisberg, C. A. *Motor Learning and Performance* (5th edition) 2011 (Champaign, IL: Human Kinetics Europe Ltd ISBN-13:978-0736069649)

Schorer, J. and Elfeink-Gemser, M. 'How good are we at predicting athletes' futures?' 2013, In. Farrow,

D., Baker, J. and MacMahon, C. (eds) *Developing Sport Expertise: Researchers and coaches put theory into practice* 2013 (Routledge pp. 30–44)

Shahbazi, M. M. and Javashi, F. 'An indirect measurement of kinematic and kinetic parameters of sprinters' 2002b *Pakistan Journal of Information and Technology* 2: pp. 228–232

Shahbazi, M. M. and Javashi, F. 'An electronic telemetry system using a laptop for investigating kinematic and kinetic studies of sprinters' 2002a, in 'Proceedings of XX ISBS Symposium' 2002, in Cacers, Spain, pp. 315–318

Singer, R. N. 'Preperformance state, routines and automaticity: What does it take to realize expertise in self-paced events?' 2002 *Journal of Sport and Exercise Psychology* 24 (4), 359–375

Slater, G. and Phillips, S. M. 'Nutrition guidelines for strength sports: sprinting, weightlifting, throwing events, and bodybuilding' 2011 *Journal of Sports Sciences*, 29 (sup1), S67–S77

Smith, G. I., Atherton, P., Reeds, D. N., Mohammed, B. S., Rankin, D., Rennie, M. J. and Mittendorfer, B. 'Omega-3 polyunsaturated fatty acids augment the muscle protein anabolic response to hyper-insulinaemia-hyperaminoacidaemia in healthy young and middle-aged men and women' 2011 *Clinical Science* 121 (6), 267–278

Smith, M. *High Performance Sprinting* 2005 (The Crowood Press Ltd ISBN-13: 978-1861267559)

Spencer, M., Bishop, D., Dawson, B. and Goodman, C. 'Physiological and metabolic responses of repeated-sprint activities' 2005 *Sports Medicine* 35 (12), 1,025–1,044

St Gibson, A. C., Lambert, E. V., Rauch, L. H., Tucker, R., Baden, D. A., Foster, C. and Noakes, T. D. 'The role of information processing between the brain and peripheral physiological systems in pacing and perception of effort' 2006 *Sports Medicine* 36 (8), 705–722

Stanton, P. and Purdam, C. 'Hamstring injuries in sprinting—the role of eccentric exercise' 1989 *Journal of Orthopaedic and Sports Physical Therapy* 10 (9), 343–349

Stellingwerff, T., Maughan, R. J. and Burke, L. M. 'Nutrition for power sports: middle-distance running, track cycling, rowing, canoeing/kayaking, and swimming' 2011 *Journal of Sports Sciences*, 29 (sup1), S79S89

Stergiou, N. *Innovative Analyses of Human Movement* 2004 (Human Kinetics Publishers)

Stone, M., Stone, M. and Sands, W. A. *Principles and Practice of Resistance Training* 2007 (Champaign, IL: Human Kinetics Europe Ltd ISBN-13:978-0880117067)

Stout, J. R., Cramer, J. T., Mielke, M., O'kroy, J., Torok, D. J. and Zoeller, R. F. 'Effects of twenty-eight days of beta-alanine and creatine monohydrate supplementation on the physical working capacity at neuromuscular fatigue threshold' 2006 *The Journal of Strength and Conditioning Research* 20 (4), 928–931

Subotnick, S. I. 'A biomechanical approach to running injuries' 1977 *Annals of the New York Academy of Sciences* 301 (1), 888–889

Syed, M. *Bounce: The Myth of Talent and the Power of Practice* 2011 (London: Fourth Estate ISBN-13:978-0007350544)

Tancred, B. and Tancred, G. *Weight Training for Sport* 1976 (London: Hodder Arnold H&S ISBN-13:978-0340344491)

Tesch, P. A., Colliander, E. B. and Kaiser, P. 'Muscle metabolism during intense, heavy-resistance exercise' 1986 *European Journal of Applied Physiology and Occupational Physiology* 55 (4), 362–366

Thijs, Y., De Clercq, D., Roosen, P. and Witvrouw, E. 'Gait-related intrinsic risk factors for patellofemoral pain in novice recreational runners' 2008 *British Journal of Sports Medicine* 42 (6), 466–471

Tiberio, D. 'The effect of excessive subtalar joint pronation on patellofemoral mechanics: a theoretical model' 1987 *Journal of Orthopaedic and Sports Physical Therapy* 9 (4), 160–165

Tibshirani, R. 'Who is the fastest man in the world?' 1997 *The American Statistician* 51 (2), 106–111

Tipton, K. D., Jeukendrup, A. E. and Hespel, P. 'Nutrition for the sprinter' 2007 *Journal of Sports Sciences*, 25 (S1), S5–S15

Toering, T. T., Elferink-Gemser, M. T., Jordet, G. and Visscher, C. 'Self-regulation and performance level of elite and non-elite youth soccer players' 2009 *Journal of Sports Sciences* 27 (14), 1,509–1,517

Ulmer, H. V. 'Concept of an extracellular regulation of muscular metabolic rate during heavy exercise in humans by psychophysiological feedback' 1996 *Experientia* 52 (5), 416–420

Vagenas, G. and Hoshizaki, T. B. 'Optimization of an asymmetrical motor skill: sprint start' 1986 *International Journal of Sport Biomechanics* 2, 29–40

van Ingen Schenau, G. J., De Koning, J. J. and De Groot, G. 'The distribution of anaerobic energy in 1000 and 4000 metre cycling bouts' 1992 *International Journal of Sports Medicine* 13 (06), 447–451

van Schenau, G. J. I., de Koning, J. J. and de Groot, G. 'Optimisation of sprinting performance in running, cycling and speed skating' 1994 *Sports Medicine* 17 (4), 259–275

Venables, M. C., Hulston, C. J., Cox, H. R. and Jeukendrup, A. E. 'Green tea extract ingestion, fat oxidation, and glucose tolerance in healthy humans' 2008 *The American Journal of Clinical Nutrition* 87 (3), 778–784

Vickers, J. N. 'Visual control when aiming at a far target' 1996 *Journal of Experimental Psychology: Human Perception and Performance* 22 (2), 324–354

Vickers, J. N. *Perception, cognition, and decision training: The quiet eye in action* 2007 (Champaign, IL: Human Kinetics)

Warden, P. *Sprinting and Hurdling: The Skills of the Game* 1989 (The Crowood Press Ltd ISBN-13: 978-1852232993)

Weinberg, R. S. and Gould, D. *Foundations of Sport and Exercise Psychology* (3rd edition) 2003 (Champaign, IL: Human Kinetics Publishers ISBN-139780736064668)

Welford, A. T. *Fundamentals of Skill* 1968 (London: Methuen)

Wells, M. *The Allan Wells Book of Sprinting* 1983 (A & C Black Publishers Ltd ISBN-13: 978-0715808436)

Weyand, P. G., Sternlight, D. B., Bellizzi, M. J. and Wright, S. 'Faster top running speeds are achieved with greater ground forces not more rapid leg movements' 2000 *Journal of Applied Physiology* 89 (5), 1,991–1,999

Wilder, R. P. and Sethi, S. 'Overuse injuries: tendinopathies, stress fractures, compartment syndrome, and shin splints' 2004 *Clinics in Sports Medicine* 23 (1), 55–81 vi. doi: 10.1016/S0278-5919(03)00085-1

Wilson, M. R. and Richards, H. In D. Collins, A. Button and H. Richards (eds.) *Performance psychology: A practitioner's guide* 2011 (pp. 177–190) (Elsevier: London)

Yeung, S. S., Suen, A. M. and Yeung, E. W. 'A prospective cohort study of hamstring injuries in competitive sprinters: preseason muscle imbalance as a possible risk factor' 2009 *British Journal of Sports Medicine* 43 (8), 589–594. doi: 10.1136/bjsm.2008.056283

Yu, B., Queen, R. M., Abbey, A. N., Liu, Y., Moorman, C. T. and Garrett, W. E. 'Hamstring muscle kinematics and activation during overground sprinting' 2008 *Journal of Biomechanics* 41(15), 3,121–3,126 doi: 10.1016 /j.jbiomech.2008.09.005

INDEX